Slim Down Now

Also by Cynthia Sass

S.A.S.S. Yourself Slim

Flat Belly Diet!

Flat Belly Diet! Cookbook

The Ultimate Diet Log

Your Diet Is Driving Me Crazy

Slim Down Now

SHED POUNDS AND INCHES
WITH REAL FOOD, REAL *FAST*

Cynthia Sass, MPH, RD

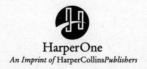

HarperOne
An Imprint of HarperCollinsPublishers

HarperOne

FIRST EDITION

Designed by Terry McGrath

Library of Congress Cataloging-in-Publication Data
Sass, Cynthia.
Slim Down Now : shed pounds and inches with real food, real fast / Cynthia Sass.
    pages cm
Includes index.
ISBN 978–0–06–231183–2
1. Reducing diets. 2. Weight loss. I. Title.
RM222.2.S2518 2015
613.2'5—dc23

                    2014035609

15 16 17 18 19 OV/RRD 10 9 8 7 6 5 4 3 2 1

For Jack Bremen
and Diane Salvagno—
thank you for always
being there for me.

Contents

[1]

Introducing the 30-Day Pulse Challenge

Most women I meet are incredibly interested in nutrition and health. They love hearing about new research on which foods will protect their heart, make their skin glow, and boost their energy. These women enjoy eating healthy, nutrient-rich foods, like greens or green juices, fruit, oats, hummus, and quinoa. But here's their dilemma: though they feel fantastic when they focus on eating healthfully, they're secretly disappointed because they don't lose weight.

As a result, most fall back into old "diet" traps like counting calories; eating processed, low-calorie, or low-fat meals; or completely cutting out carbs, including fruits, whole grains, and even many vegetables. Yes, they start losing weight again, but they also feel drained of energy, irritable, and plagued by nagging hunger. They also struggle with the unpleasant side effects of dieting, like headaches, trouble sleeping, constipation, and a dull appearance. Yet these women push on because they're just not ready to give up on getting slimmer, and they don't know how else to get there.

This book offers another path. It's a simple yet powerful meal-building strategy that will allow you to enjoy healthy foods, feel satisfied and energetic, *and* lose weight—all at the same time. This intersection of weight loss and cutting-edge nutrition is what so many women tell me they desperately want to find but can't. I will get you there.

Here's what I'm offering: a 30-day challenge during which you'll take a break from your usual weight-loss methods and adopt an entirely new approach to food, health, and weight management.

In one month's time, you'll learn exactly how to eat the healthiest foods on the planet—including one special group I've chosen as the star of this plan—in the right amounts, in the right balance, and at the right times. My strategy will allow you to feel amazing *and* get the weight-loss results you want, and it's far simpler than you might think.

My plan has two parts: the four-day Rapid Pulse and the twenty-six-day Daily Pulse. The cornerstone of both is a unique and awesome class of protein-rich carbs called pulses: the edible goodies that come from plants in the legume family, which include lentils, chickpeas, and many varieties of beans. (The term *pulse* is popular in Europe, Latin America, and India but is less well known in the United States.) Scientists have published an amazing amount of research on pulses, and I'm convinced that making pulses a daily staple is the key to weight loss and good health. In my opinion, pulses are the single most underrated superfood.

The latest science shows that just as not all calories are created equal, not all carbs are created equal. Pulses have been shown to boost calorie and fat burning, whittle away belly fat, enhance fullness (to curb appetite and prevent snack attacks), and support all-day feelings of energy. What's more, they protect your heart, lower your risk for type 2 diabetes and cancer, and improve your overall nutrient intake. They're also gluten free, they don't trigger allergies, and they're affordable and readily available. I know you'll find them to be incredibly satisfying, rich in flavor, and versatile! I bet you already love at least one healthy dish that contains a pulse, like hummus or White Bean and Kale Soup. But you probably don't know half of the amazing things you can do with pulses. You'll learn about their incredible weight loss and health benefits in chapter 4, and you won't believe the creative ways I've built them into this plan.

During the Rapid Pulse, you'll make just one quick and easy recipe: a pudding, which you'll eat three times a day. I'm confident that you'll fall in love with its flavor (you actually get to choose from three delicious options) and thick, creamy texture. In fact, I bet you'll want to keep making my unique pudding recipe long after the Rapid Pulse is over. Even my hubby, who's hardly a health nut, regularly asks me to make it, and kids love it—even though I've snuck a pulse (black or white beans) into the recipe! Now, before you think "No way!" and snap this book shut, trust me. You won't even know the beans are in there. (Ever tried black bean brownies or Chinese red bean ice cream? Both are delicious!)

This Rapid Pulse phase is ultra simple, because the pudding can be whipped up in five minutes and enjoyed chilled or warmed. Or you can add water and ice to turn it into a smoothie. Plus, you can make two days' worth of servings ahead of time, so you only need to prepare food twice in four days. Sound easy? It is. The repetition of the single recipe serves a purpose, as I explain in chapter 2, and I chose the ingredients carefully to maximize your four-day weight loss without leaving you feeling hungry.

The Rapid Pulse will help you shed up to eight pounds in four days, so you'll be well on your way to your weight goal. Then you'll transition to the Daily Pulse, which will keep you losing straight through day thirty. As you may guess from the name, this phase includes one serving of pulse each day. That's the secret sauce in this plan. But it's not the only critical component. You'll incorporate the pulse serving into a simple meal-building strategy that doesn't require you to count calories, points, or grams or memorize any complicated numbers or charts. The power of the Daily Pulse comes from enjoying a specific combination of three food groups in the right portions at the right times. Once you master this strategy, you'll discover how simple it is, how much sense it makes, and how easy it will be to apply no matter where you are. The final essential component of the plan is learning precisely how to add other healthy, carb-rich foods—like sweet potatoes, spaghetti squash, bananas, and quinoa—to your meals without compromising weight loss. I refer to these foods as *energy accessories*.

From day five through day thirty, you'll enjoy hearty, filling dishes, like savory quiche, chicken cacciatore, shrimp scampi, lemony hummus, lentil soup, and oven-roasted potatoes. And I've dedicated an entire chapter to desserts! You'll get to savor luscious brownie bites, vanilla cinnamon chocolate truffles, frozen cherry coconut pops, and my favorite, pumpkin-spice mini muffins. Incorporating these indulgences into the 30-day challenge will give you sweet treats to look forward to and help you stay on track. So instead of battling to stay on an ultra-strict "diet"—a battle you're destined to lose—you'll maintain a consistent eating pattern all month long.

Meanwhile, you won't be running yourself ragged trying to maintain an intense workout regimen. Part of this 30-day challenge is letting go of traditional notions of exercise. You'll adopt a whole new approach to movement that doesn't feel tedious or punishing and is based on a less-is-more philosophy that's backed by research. For countless people I talk to, the forms of physical activity associated with weight loss, like running, boot-camp classes, and elliptical machines, are a major turn off. So people skip their workouts altogether or they fizzle out fast, rebounding right back to inactivity.

I'm going to help you find ways to move that feel fun. You'll actually look forward to being active over the next thirty days! I'll also share the science that explains why *less* exercise, rather than more, can actually set you up to be more successful at weight loss. And I'll reveal how to strategically remove the two biggest obstacles that get in the way of being active: stress and time constraints. When you ditch the no pain, no gain idea, you'll not only lose weight but also find yourself healthier and in a better mood.

The final critical element of my plan is meditation—just five short minutes a day! Meditation is essentially yoga for your mind, and if you've never tried it, you're in for a real treat. I'll show you how to make meditation part of your daily routine, but don't worry: you don't need to light incense, chant, repeat a mantra, sit cross-legged, or carve out much time from your day. And the rewards will be tremendous. Practicing meditation daily will lower your stress hormone levels, reduce inflammation (a known accelerator of aging and disease), curb your desire to eat impulsively, and increase your motivation to be active. What's more, when you meditate, you'll feel calmer and happier, and you'll experience a clarity of mind that allows you to better absorb new information (like the contents of this book!).

By day thirty-one, my meal-building strategy will feel like your new normal, allowing you to either maintain your weight loss or keep shedding pounds if you haven't yet reached your goal. More important, you'll have a new outlook on life, because you'll have found the solution to losing weight while feeling fabulous, not famished. While your friends, family members, or coworkers start yet another low-carb, low-cal, complicated, or strict diet, you'll be enjoying omelets with potatoes, fruit smoothies, satay with noodles, and desserts! Your energy will soar while you drop dress and jean sizes.

Are you ready to end a chaotic relationship with food and finally find freedom from the struggle between getting thin and feeling healthy? Get set to ditch "dieting," embrace optimal health, and reach your dream weight. Get ready to have it all.

My Story

Sandy Pinzon, age 34

Lost 14.8 pounds and 12.5 inches

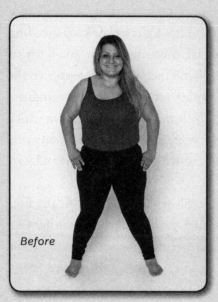

Before

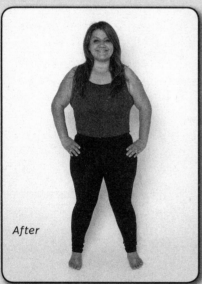

After

Before this meal plan my eating was very unorganized. There were days I'd forget to eat, and on other days I felt like I ate all day but just didn't feel full or satisfied. This 30-day challenge taught me that I am consistently capable of making healthy choices every day. I also learned that it's possible to eat smaller portions and actually get filled! Never did I think that my last meal would be at 5 or 6 pm, and I would be content for the rest of the evening! The meals are light but also filling, and after getting the hang of the plan, I never felt hungry other than at my regular mealtimes.

I am *very* thankful for this opportunity because I didn't have to kill myself to shed the excess pounds. My clothes are loose, I've received several compliments from friends who have noticed the weight loss, and I feel a lot healthier in general. It feels so good to "eat clean."

20 21 22 23 24 25 26 27 28 29 30 31 32 33 34 35 36 37

My fourteen-year-old daughter followed the plan with me. The wardrobe metaphor was so easy that she knew what was needed for each meal. The wardrobe concept was what I liked most about the plan. It made it very easy to understand and follow. Sometimes when I didn't have time to plan a meal or was out of the house, I'd just think back to the wardrobe concept, and I was able to create a light and filling meal. In fact, even though this has been my busiest time of the year at work, I've been able to stick with this plan. That says a lot.

I would tell any woman who is considering this plan to definitely try it! You'll learn how to eat in moderation and to how to eat healthier and cleaner. Also, with this plan you don't feel hungry and you still see results (not feeling hungry has been the biggest selling point for me!). I am amazed with the results in such a short time—and I barely had any time to exercise!

I've tried so many things in the past to lose weight without getting much of a result. This is the first time in years I've actually eaten correctly, and I definitely plan to continue eating this way. I want this to be my new way of life!

21 22 23 24 25 26 27 28 29 30 31 32 33 34 35 36 37 3

[2]

The Rapid Pulse

Most "diets" have an initial phase that involves serious deprivation, even downright starvation—modes your body and mind strongly rebel against. You might subsist for days or weeks on plain chicken and steamed spinach, chalky shakes, or bitter detox drinks.

Forget all that! During my plan's kick-start phase, the Rapid Pulse, you get to indulge in thick, rich pudding. For four days, you'll eat a delicious, satisfying pudding three times a day. Along the way, you'll shed up to 8 pounds, regain normal appetite regulation, and reboot your metabolism. Even better, you'll find the confidence and momentum to transition to the next step in your weight-loss journey.

There are three puddings to choose from—Ginger Fig, Mango Vanilla, and Dark Chocolate—and each one contains a short list of exceptional ingredients, including beans. (Yes, beans in a pudding! Not to worry—you won't taste them.) You can enjoy the pudding cold or warm, and you can whip it up in just five minutes—no cooking involved. You can even blend up two days' worth of pudding in advance and pop it in the fridge, so you need only prepare food twice in four days. Or if you prefer, you can add water and ice to transform the pudding into a smoothie.

You need to choose just *one* of these three puddings to commit to for all four days. In other words, you *cannot* eat the ginger pudding on day one, then switch to mango on day two, or eat a variety of the three puddings over the four days. This is because the repetition of eating the same exact pudding daily for all four days is an important aspect of how this phase helps you lose weight.

If you really love chocolate, choosing the chocolate version may be a no-brainer. However, I would encourage you to choose the one you think you'll enjoy most, especially since you'll be eating it exclusively for four days! If you're not sure which one you think you'll like best, try making one batch of each as you prepare to start this plan. This "taste test" will ensure that you choose the right version for your taste preferences.

Now, I know what you may be thinking: *I like pudding, but can I really eat the same pudding three times a day for four days in a row?*

Absolutely. In fact, the women who have already lost weight on this plan have enjoyed it greatly. And if you're like most of my clients, four days of pudding is exactly what you need. Here's what I mean: When my clients come to me, they're typically feeling frustrated by their inability to lose weight and exhausted from the demands of everyday life. They're eager for a simple weight-loss solution. They're not in the mood to memorize food lists, track fat or carb grams, or follow complex rules. They just want to lose weight without feeling overwhelmed or deprived. Many women have told me "Sometimes I think it would just be easier to stay fat," though in their hearts, they don't want to give up.

If you can relate, you'll be happy to know I designed the Rapid Pulse phase to be incredibly easy, effective, and burden free. This brief phase represents a turning point in your relationship with food and your body.

You'll introduce your body to a weight-loss superfood—pulses—that will become a daily staple. And after just four days, you'll feel newly empowered—ready to embark on a path to weight loss that feels sane, sustainable, and satisfying.

That's one reason I call this phase the Rapid Pulse: it allows you to shed pounds quickly. Another reason is that everything about this kick start is streamlined. You rely on one simple recipe, which takes just five minutes to make. Rapid meals, rapid results.

The *pulse* part of the name has a dual meaning as well. Pulses are the edible parts of plants in the legume family. Pulses include lentils, chickpeas, and a wide variety of beans. During the Rapid Pulse, your pudding base is one of these goodies: black or white beans.

But *pulse* also signifies life. Your pulse is the rhythmic beat of your arteries as blood is propelled through them. That's fitting, because in addition to promoting heart health, this entire plan—the Rapid Pulse and the Daily Pulse combined—is designed to enhance your life or, if you've been struggling with stress, low energy, and an on-and-off diet cycle, make you feel as if you've come back to life.

So let's get right to it! In the following sections, I'll give you the three pudding recipes and the simple Rapid Pulse rules, along with a shopping list that covers all four days. I'll explain why you won't get bored eating just one dish, and why I have based this entire kick start on a pudding. I'll also answer other pressing questions, like "What's so special about the pudding ingredients?" and "What will I be able to drink on the plan?"

The Pudding Recipes

Here's how to make the thick, delicious pudding that will sustain you for the next four days. Note that it's important to make the pudding one batch at a time. Even a high-powered food processor may not blend the ingredients well enough when multiple batches are made at once.

Ginger Fig Pulse Pudding

SERVES 1

½ cup unsweetened coconut milk (from the dairy case, not a can)
2 tablespoons chia seeds (black or white)
½ cup fresh banana slices (approximately 1 small to medium banana)
¼ cup canned black beans, drained and rinsed
2 small to medium dried black Mission figs, stems removed
½ teaspoon fresh ginger, grated and peeled
1 tablespoon unsweetened shredded or flaked coconut

In a blender or food processor, combine the coconut milk, chia seeds, banana, black beans, figs, and ginger. Blend until the mixture is smooth. Transfer it to a tall glass or bowl and top it with the coconut.

To serve chilled, refrigerate the pudding for at least 30 minutes.

To serve warm, microwave the pudding on high for 1 minute (1½ minutes if the pudding has been in the fridge). Test it with your finger to make sure it's not too hot before eating.

Mango Vanilla Pulse Pudding

SERVES 1

½ cup unsweetened coconut milk (from the dairy case, not a can)
2 tablespoons chia seeds (black or white)
½ cup fresh yellow mango (the yellow-skinned variety, not the green-skinned variety)
¼ cup canned white beans, drained and rinsed (includes navy, great northern, or cannellini)
½ teaspoon ground cinnamon
½ teaspoon pure vanilla extract
1 tablespoon honey (optional)

In a blender or food processor, combine the coconut milk, chia seeds, mango, white beans, cinnamon, and vanilla extract. Taste the mixture and add up to 1 tablespoon of honey if desired. Blend until it is smooth. Transfer it to a tall glass or bowl.

To serve chilled, refrigerate the pudding for at least 30 minutes.

To serve warm, microwave the pudding on high for 1 minute (1½ minutes if the pudding has been in the fridge). Test it with your finger to make sure it's not too hot before eating.

Dark Chocolate Pulse Pudding

....

SERVES 1

½ cup unsweetened coconut milk (from the dairy case, not a can)

2 tablespoons chia seeds (black or white)

3 medium pitted dates, minced, soaked in 1 tablespoon water for at least
    10 minutes

2 tablespoons unsweetened cocoa powder

¼ cup canned white beans, drained and rinsed (includes navy, great northern,
    or cannellini)

1 teaspoon pure vanilla extract

1 tablespoon honey (optional)

In a blender or food processor, combine the coconut milk, chia seeds, dates, cocoa powder, white beans, and vanilla extract. Taste the mixture and add up to 1 tablespoon of honey if desired. Blend until it is smooth. Transfer it to a tall glass or bowl.

To serve chilled, refrigerate the pudding for at least 30 minutes.

To serve warm, microwave the pudding on high for 1 minute (1½ minute if the pudding has been in the fridge). Test it with your finger to make sure it's not too hot before eating.

Smoothie Option: If you dislike the texture of pudding, you can turn your pudding recipe into a smoothie! Just add ⅓ cup water and 4 to 5 ice cubes. Be sure to do this right before you're ready to start sipping. In other words, don't make the smoothies in advance. For the smoothie option, you can either take a premade pudding, add water and ice, and whip it in a blender just before drinking, or make a fresh smoothie using the ingredients for one batch of pudding, blending them with water and ice just before drinking.

When to Eat the Pudding

For each of the next four days, eat three servings of pudding, the first within an hour of waking up and the other two servings four to five hours apart. For example

    Pudding 1: 9 A.M.

    Pudding 2: 1 P.M.

    Pudding 3: 6 P.M.

or

Pudding 1: 8:00 A.M.

Pudding 2: 12:00 P.M.

Pudding 3: 5:00 P.M.

or

Pudding 1: 7:00 A.M.

Pudding 2: 12:00 P.M.

Pudding 3: 5:00 P.M.

Take as much time as you'd like to eat each serving, and if you feel full, you don't have to finish it! One reason I chose a pudding is that enjoying pudding at a leisurely pace is intuitive—and eating slowly has been shown to boost feelings of fullness and enjoyment (see page 206). Some of the women who tested the Rapid Pulse reported taking thirty minutes to finish one serving of pudding, which allowed them to feel like they were eating far more than a single portion. Eating a little at a time and stashing it back in the fridge is just fine. So if you'd like, you could eat half of a pudding serving every two to two and a half hours. For example

- First half of pudding 1: 7 A.M.
- Second half of pudding 1: 9 A.M.
- First half of pudding 2: 12 P.M.
- Second half of pudding 2: 2 P.M.
- First half of pudding 3: 5 P.M.
- Second half of pudding 3: 7 P.M.

Or you could go halfsies with one or two of the puddings rather than all three. Just be sure to finish each pudding by the five-hour mark. In other words, don't save halves and move them into other time blocks. To keep your metabolism revved, energy supported, and appetite in check, your body needs a steady supply of nutrients spread throughout the day. Going long stretches without eating and then eating a lot in one sitting is antagonistic to how your body optimally operates. In fact, it's exactly how sumo wrestlers purposely gain weight!

THE RAPID PULSE RULES

- Eat three pudding servings a day for four days.
- Eat the first serving within one hour of waking up, and space the remaining two no less than four hours and no more than five hours apart.
- It's okay to not finish the pudding.
- It's okay to take as much time as you need to eat each serving, as long as you don't "save" a portion and move it into another time block (unless you're doing halfsies).
- If you really dislike the texture of pudding, you can turn your pudding recipe into a smoothie. Just add ⅓ cup water and 4 to 5 ice cubes.
- Drink only the allowed beverages, listed on page 33.
- Complete a five-minute meditation, what I like to refer to as a "mind massage," each day. (I explain this starting on page 46.)
- If you exercise during the Rapid Pulse, wait sixty to ninety minutes after eating a pudding serving. Do not engage in intense exercise, or work out for more than an hour each day.

Why You Won't Get Bored on Pudding Alone

In addition to counseling private clients, I'm a nutrition and health writer, and it's my job to stay abreast of research and trends. Part of my morning routine is to make my coffee, flip open my laptop, and scour the latest studies. During this ritual, I'll occasionally experience a eureka moment: A study will pop up that completely jibes with what I'm seeing in my one-on-one counseling work. In those instances, I know I've hit upon something significant.

One such realization struck me after reading a study about how apps like Instagram affect how we experience our food. Researchers at Brigham Young University recruited over two hundred volunteers to look at photos of food, then eat, then rate how much they enjoyed their snack. When the volunteers ate foods similar to what they'd viewed, they reported enjoying the foods less than when they ate foods they hadn't seen. Why? The scientists concluded that by viewing the photos, the volunteers had already "experienced" the food, which triggered a sense of "doneness." This intuitively makes sense, because we eat with our eyes as well as our stomachs, and our culture is so visually oriented. But what really hit me was how this research could be used in entirely opposing ways: to enhance the enjoyment of food or to trigger satiety and diminish the desire to eat when you're trying to lose weight.

According to this research, if I was preparing a Thanksgiving dinner, I wouldn't want my guests to jump on Pinterest, Instagram, or Flickr before attending my feast, because viewing fluffy mounds of mashed potatoes and glistening pumpkin pies online might presate their palates, thereby diminishing how much they enjoy my dishes. On the other hand, if I was attending a dinner and didn't want to leave with that overly stuffed feeling many of us regretfully experience on holidays, logging on to those photo-sharing sites would be a savvy way to help rein in my appetite.

This intriguing research offers new insight into *satiation,* which is the drop in enjoyment with repeated consumption. And that's where the pudding comes in. If you've ever bought something new, whether a video game or a pair of shoes, you've surely experienced the sense of wonderment attached to the newness. But over time the novelty fades. The more you play the game, the less exciting it becomes; those must-have shoes eventually become just another pair in your collection. The same is true for food, and scientists even have a term for it: habituation. In a nutshell, *habituation* means that eating a food repeatedly makes you lose interest, and you will naturally eat less.

To test this theory, scientists from the University at Buffalo and the University of Vermont randomly assigned obese and nonobese women to eat macaroni and cheese five times, either once a day for five days or once a week for five weeks. No matter what the volunteers weighed, the women offered mac 'n' cheese daily ate progressively less, whereas the women offered the dish weekly ate progressively more. Makes sense, right? The more often you eat something without taking a break, the less exciting it becomes—kind of a "been there, done that" phenomenon.

Sameness is key. The scientists point out that for habituation to kick in, the meals must be identical. In other words, eating pizza daily won't prompt you to eat less pizza if the toppings change. Even small variations stimulate the senses in new ways, much like how playing the same old video game with a new challenger can reignite your interest.

This eat, repeat, and lose interest syndrome is one reason I've chosen a single recipe for the Rapid Pulse phase. I'm confident you'll get through four days of eating nothing but your chosen pudding. In fact, I bet you'll want to do it again in the future. But I also know that by day four, you'll be plenty tired of pudding. And in my experience, that's a very good thing, because the simplicity and repetition of this phase will give you a whole new sense of appetite regulation.

When most of my clients begin a kick start, they're either completely disconnected from hunger and fullness cues or they feel perpetually hungry. The Rapid Pulse is like hitting the reset button. Within four days, you'll begin to reconnect with a normal sense of hunger and fullness, and reboot your metabolism so that you maximize the number of calories your body burns. (See What to Expect During the Rapid Pulse on page 45.)

Habituation, however, isn't the only reason I developed these puddings. Another is simplicity. When I set out to create the ultimate kick start, I began with three different daily meals: one breakfast, one lunch, and one dinner. I intended for this pattern to be repeated daily for four days. This approach has worked for many of my clients, and the meals were basic, but my gut kept telling me, *Keep it simple, simple, simple, simple.* And when I went to my local market to shop for the groceries, even I felt overwhelmed by the number of items needed for just four days. Waiting in line at the checkout, I thought about all the women who feel stuck and overwhelmed and just need to be able to think, *Yes, I can do that!*

So I streamlined. After much consideration, I decided an optimal kick start would have to be based on a single dish that would

- taste so delicious you could enjoy eating it for four consecutive days;
- require a short list of ingredients, few steps, and no stove or oven;
- be easy to make ahead and eat at home or take on the go;
- taste yummy either chilled or warmed up;
- be free from common allergens and irritants, such as dairy, gluten, soy, eggs, and nuts;
- contain protein and be suitable for vegans and vegetarians; and
- provide a texture and contain ingredients that support weight loss, optimize energy, and promote fullness and satisfaction.

Of my original meals, one was the clear standout: pudding. So my next step was to test it on my unsuspecting hubby, Jack. Jack is used to taste-testing my recipes, and he's completely honest with his feedback. I once developed a recipe for a healthy meal makeover in a magazine. I was happy with how the casserole came out and proudly handed it to him on a plate. He took one bite and said, "Eh, this tastes too healthy. I know you probably like it, but I wouldn't ask you to make it for me" (my true litmus test). So I went back into the kitchen, tweaked it, and finally earned his thumbs-up. I have to admit, the final recipe was a lot better. So Jack is like my in-house, one-man panel of judges.

As he was working on his computer, I approached him with the Ginger Fig Pulse Pudding and simply said, "Can you please try this and tell me what you think?" Normally he takes a bite or spoonful, offers his feedback, and goes back to work. But this time he asked if he could eat the whole thing. A smile exploded across my face and I said, "Sure!" He could tell the pudding contained banana and coconut, two of his favorite foods, as well as ginger (one of my staple ingredients), but his favorite part was the thick texture. When he asked if I could make it again and told me he couldn't finish it because it was so filling, I knew I had a winner. After I took the bowl away, I couldn't hold it in anymore. I had to tell him that the secret ingredient was . . . drumroll please . . . black beans. I wish I could have snapped a photo of his face. It took a second to register, then his brow furrowed slightly, then "Aw, really? Why did you make me eat that?" But a few minutes later he was over it and said he would eat it again!

My next tester was my sister, whom I trust wholeheartedly. Diane always offers honest, constructive criticism with a kindness and sincerity that gives me the warm fuzzies, even if what she says means I need to go back to the drawing board. I held my breath as I waited for her feedback, because she was making the pudding herself, fully knowing what went into it. When she said "I love it!" I practically jumped for joy! Like Jack, she loved the texture as well as the tropical banana-coconut combination. She also thought it was fun to make. And though she was skeptical of the beans, she admitted that if she didn't know they were in there, she never would have guessed. She also suspected they were the reason the pudding was so filling. "It filled me up the way a black bean salad does," she said, "but it's pudding!" Bingo! When it came time to test the Rapid Pulse with real women, I found that some had a strong dislike of ginger, so I decided to add two more flavor options—mango vanilla and dark chocolate. Between the three, I bet you'll find one that suits your taste buds. And you can incorporate any pudding you like as a dessert option during the Daily Pulse.

Why Pudding?

I think my sister hit the nail on the head. Pudding is heavenly. There's just something blissful about repeatedly dipping in, and each spoonful is a sensory sensation. It's comfort in a cup.

But that's not the only reason I chose pudding as the signature dish of this phase. As I explained earlier, pudding is something you intuitively eat slowly. What's more, pudding's thickness prompts eaters to perceive it as particularly filling. How hungry or full we feel is, of course, influenced by the type of foods we eat and the sizes of our portions, but research shows it's also affected by the thickness of our foods. For example, in a University of Sussex study, researchers asked volunteers to rate how filling they expected various thick, creamy drinks to be. The volunteers did this by identifying how much solid food they thought they would need to eat to experience the same degree of fullness. The researchers concluded that thickness, but not creaminess, influenced the expectation that a drink would suppress hunger over time.

In two other studies, thicker drinks were found to suppress actual hunger (not just anticipated hunger, as in the Sussex study) more than thinner versions of beverages with the same calorie levels. A thick texture, it appears, is a characteristic we associate with an extended period of fullness.

When you make the pudding for the first time, you'll see just how thick it is. And as you dip in your spoon, you'll not only expect to feel full, but you actually will feel as full as if you'd eaten a solid meal. That's an important reason the Rapid Pulse is so effective.

Also important: the thickness of the pudding forces you to eat at a more leisurely pace. If you tend to gobble down your food, as most of us do, the Rapid Pulse will compel you to s-l-o-w down. This change will help you succeed over the next four days. And once slower eating becomes second nature, your new eating pace has the power to end mindless eating and overeating forever.

Research shows that speed eating curtails the release of hormones that trigger feelings of fullness, so you overeat without even realizing it. On the flip side, slow eaters take in about four times fewer calories per minute and experience a higher level of satiety, even when they eat less food. Simply by eating pudding, you'll slow down. Or if you choose to make the pudding into a smoothie, you can sip it slowly. And the daily five-minute mind massage meditation (on page 46) you'll begin during this phase will decelerate you even more during meals and beyond. (For more about the remarkable impact of meditation, see chapter 7.)

Beans? In a Pudding? Really?

So you know why I created a pudding. But did I really have to put beans in it? It may seem unconventional here in the West, but bean puddings are actually quite common in other parts of the globe. The first time I tried one was at a Vietnamese deli in New York City. At the time, *bánh mì,* or Vietnamese sandwiches, were all the rage, so Jack and I ventured out to a little place that was supposed to be the best in Manhattan. To my surprise, the menu included not only hoagies and summer rolls but also pudding, made with chickpeas or black-eyed peas. I chose the chickpea, and it was

TAKE A BREAK FROM CALORIE COUNTS

As you may notice, I didn't include the calorie counts for the puddings here, and even if you have access to a program that can compute it, I encourage you to maintain the mystery. As I'll show throughout this book, the latest research illustrates that calories aren't the be-all, end-all for weight control, and not all calories are created equal. A lot of factors impact what happens to calories after they're absorbed; these include a food's nutrient profile (the amount of antioxidants, fiber, protein, and so on), aroma, flavor, texture, and rate of digestion. So, even at the same calorie level or lower, a processed pudding that's made with refined sugar and is missing the pulse and fruit of the Rapid Pulse puddings would have a very different impact on your metabolism, blood sugar and insulin response, appetite, and weight. Even the type of carbs in a dish and the nutrients they're combined with are far more important than the total number of carb grams. So forego the calculations, and focus on quality and balance, the real keys to success and satisfaction.

delicious! (Nothing like hummus, by the way.) Shortly after that, I visited Japan and was fascinated by the use of adzuki beans in desserts, from ice cream and mooncakes to *yōkan,* a popular jellied bean treat served in blocks or slices. The idea of using beans in sweet rather than savory recipes stuck with me, so when I began developing my *Slim Down Now* recipes, bean pudding was the very first idea that popped into my head. I love it so much, I often make a portion for myself for breakfast, chilled in the summer months and warmed up in the fall and winter.

Are Three Meals a Day Enough?

The eating plans in my previous two books included four meals a day, but I have found, both in my private practice and in my correspondence with readers, that for many people, only three meals are necessary, particularly if the meals are spaced no more than five hours apart. This is especially true for women over forty, those with sedentary jobs, and people who are only able to fit in exercise a few times a week. The truth is, it's much, much easier to add food to a plan than it is to take food away. And based on my experience and the available research, I believe that eating three square meals a day is plenty for most adults, and I've found that it's the best place to start.

Consider, for example, a recent Dutch study published in the *British Journal of Nutrition*. The study divided women into two groups offered the same number of calories. One group received just two meals per day, breakfast and dinner, spaced eight and a half hours apart. The second group ate three daily meals—breakfast, lunch, and dinner—spaced four hours apart. The three-a-day group reported feeling more full over twenty-four hours than the two-a-day group. They also burned more fat, particularly in the evening. This may make you wonder if a fourth, fifth, or sixth meal would be even better, but the answer is no.

When University of Colorado scientists compared breaking the same amount of food into six rather than three meals, they found no difference in metabolism, meaning both groups experienced similar rates of calorie and fat burning. But there was a downside to eating more frequently: the six-meal-a-day group experienced more hunger and a greater overall desire to eat.

Why Black and White Beans?

While my husband's big question was "Did you really have to put beans in it?" my sister's was "Why black and white beans?" Well, when I set out to create this plan, choosing black and white beans felt completely fitting for multiple reasons. For one thing, the kick-start phase of a plan is black and white, metaphorically speaking. It's about finding an approach that's ultra-simple, all laid out for you, and short term. If you've been struggling to find something that works and doesn't make you miserable, approaching this first step toward weight loss in a black-and-white fashion is the best way to garner success.

But beyond philosophy, I knew from the latest science that foods that are literally black and white in color are loaded with potent health-promoting substances. We've all read about the beneficial antioxidants and phytochemicals in green leafy vegetables or brightly colored berries. But impressive research has found that the antioxidants associated with foods that are naturally black and white—foods we normally do not seek out—are just as beneficial for weight loss and enhancing health.

Black foods, such as black beans and Mission figs, which are striking in color and enticing in flavor, are also loaded with natural disease-fighting chemicals. These naturally raven-colored foods contain substances called anthocyanins, a type of phenolic compound (remember that term) specifically in the flavonoid group. You may have heard about anthocyanins because they're found in superfoods such as tea, wine, and cocoa.

In a recent Japanese study, researchers fed groups of mice a fatty diet with and without anthocyanins. The mice given the protective pigments, unlike the other mice, didn't gain body weight or body fat and did not experience a spike in blood sugar, insulin, and blood fats. Researchers concluded that anthocyanins act as a "functional food component" that may help prevent obesity and diabetes.

Some of anthocyanins' effectiveness is surely related to their impact on inflammation. Stubbing your toe is a classic example of "good" inflammation. The throbbing pain is accompanied by swelling and an immune-system response, which promotes healing. But when low-grade inflammation occurs at the cellular level, it creates a cascade of problems, from premature aging to cell damage and disease. We now know this type of chronic inflammation is tied to heart disease, osteoporosis, arthritis, brain disorders, diabetes, and obesity. To assess levels of "bad" inflammation, scientists look at markers in the blood, including one called C-reactive protein, or CRP. A twenty-four-week study, published in the journal *Nutrition, Metabolism, and Cardiovascular Diseases,* found that anthocyanins slashed CRP levels by 22 percent in adults with high cholesterol. Also, the subjects' "good" (HDL) cholesterol levels rose by 14 percent, and their "bad" (LDL) levels dropped by 10 percent.

Naturally white foods, which I find to be quite elegant, also offer anti-inflammatory benefits. Banana, ginger, white beans, and coconut each contain those natural substances called phenolic compounds (that term I asked you to remember from the previous page). A fascinating U.K. study from the University of Leeds found that phenolic compounds inhibited or blunted the absorption of glucose (sugar) from the digestive tract into the bloodstream, improving blood sugar and insulin regulation. This link is an important finding, not only for diabetes prevention and management but also for weight control. When glucose enters your bloodstream, your blood sugar level rises and insulin is secreted. This hormone's job is to bring sugar to your cells, to be used for fuel. But if blood sugar rises too quickly and insulin spikes, your cells have access to more sugar than they can burn or use, and the surplus gets socked away as fat. When this happens, your blood sugar level drops again, causing your energy level to plummet and triggering your appetite once more. So at the same time you're storing body fat, you're already feeling hungry again.

Spanish researchers also found evidence that phenolic compounds may explain many of the health benefits of the Mediterranean diet. Compared to study subjects who ate Mediterranean meals without phenolic compounds, those who ate Mediterranean meals with these compounds experienced better blood vessel relaxation and improved blood flow, which reduce stress on the heart. Better blood flow also means better delivery of oxygen and nutrients to every one of your cells, from head to toe. Another Spanish study, which tracked over eight hundred seniors, found that over a twelve-year period, those with the highest intake of phenolics had a 30 percent lower death rate.

Based on these and other studies linking antioxidants to mechanisms in the body that control weight and body composition, I am quite convinced that nutrition science research will continue to reveal their roles and benefits. But in addition to their antioxidants, there are other health and nutritional reasons I selected the key ingredients that make up the Rapid Pulse puddings.

Simple Sensational Ingredients

Chia Seeds

Remember the famous song from the pet plant commercials, "Chi, chi, chi, chia . . ."? In those days, few people thought of chia as a food, but in recent years, chia seeds have exploded in popularity—and I have to admit, I'm quite taken with them. These tiny oval seeds are rich in a type of omega-3 fatty acid called alpha-linolenic acid, or ALA. Several studies have examined the relationship between dietary ALA intake and health. In a study of more than seventy-six thousand U.S. women followed for ten years, those with the highest ALA intakes had a risk of fatal heart disease 45 percent lower than women with the lowest intakes of ALA. Another study, in more than forty-five thousand U.S. men followed for fourteen years, found that each 1-gram-per-day increase in ALA intake was tied to a 16 percent reduction in heart disease risk. In those who ate little or no seafood, the risk protection soared to 47 percent.

A recent study looked at the effect of chia seeds, technically known as *Salvia hispanica,* on post-meal blood sugar levels. Ground and whole seeds were equally effective at reducing postmeal blood glucose (for more about why this is so critical for weight control, see page 243). Chia seeds also contain the phenolic compounds I described on page 22, and the 2-tablespoon portion you add to each pudding packs a whopping 40 percent of the minimum daily recommended fiber intake.

One of my favorite properties of chia seeds is the gel-like texture they create, due to their ability to soak up about twelve times their weight in fluid. This superstar ingredient is another reason the Rapid Pulse puddings are so thick and satisfying.

What to look for:

These days you can buy chia seeds at many mainstream grocery stores, but if your local market doesn't carry them, you can find them online. They're typically sold in resealable bags and come in white and black varieties. I prefer the aesthetic appeal of black myself, unless I'm using them in a recipe that would be better suited to white. For any pudding you choose, either color is fine. Just make sure the only ingredient in the bag is whole (not ground) chia seeds. After opening the bag, store it in a cool, dry place, away from sunlight.

Tip:

If you ever spill chia seeds in your kitchen, try not to get them wet. This happened to me once, and I had quite a sticky mess on my hands!

Coconut

The Rapid Pulse puddings each contain coconut milk, and the Ginger Fig version also includes shredded coconut. Coconut has historically been associated with decadence and weight gain. But like chia seeds, it has recently become popular as a health food. What's the bottom line? Coconut gets a clear thumbs-up.

Several studies have found that the fat in coconut aids weight loss. It belongs to a group of saturated fats called medium-chain triglycerides, or MCTs, which are metabolized in a unique way. More research confirms that not all saturated fats are bad for you. The type found in coconut has actually been shown to raise HDL (good) cholesterol and promote the loss of belly fat.

In one twelve-week study, Brazilian researchers tested the effects of adding about 1 ounce daily of either soybean oil or coconut oil to the diets of women who were instructed to follow a balanced eating plan and walk for fifty minutes a day. Body weights decreased in both groups, but only the coconut oil eaters experienced a reduction in waist measurements. At the end of the study, they also had higher levels of good HDL cholesterol and lower LDL to HDL ratios.

Another study, published in the *European Journal of Clinical Nutrition,* found that over eight weeks, MCTs reduced body weight, body fat, waist size, and belly fat in women with high triglycerides, a type of blood fat. MCTs have also been shown to boost calorie and fat burning. Plus, coconut provides antioxidants similar to those in berries, grapes, and dark chocolate.

What to look for:

Look for unsweetened coconut milk, either in the dairy case or in shelf-stable quarts. It's often sold next to other plant-based milk substitutes, like almond milk. Do not buy coconut milk sold in cans, even light versions. These varieties contain much less water, packing as much as ten times the calories per cup. Your unsweetened coconut milk should provide roughly 45 to 60 calories, 4 or 5 grams of fat, 1 or 2 grams of carbohydrate, and no protein per cup. A fortified version that contains added nutrients, like vitamin B_{12} is fine. Just be sure it's unsweetened.

If you choose to make the Ginger Fig Pulse Pudding, when shopping for shredded coconut, turn the package over and read the ingredient list. The only words you should see are "natural coconut," "dehydrated coconut," or "unsulfured coconut." Either shredded or flaked is fine. I love the way flakes look, but I also like to stir finer shreds into my pudding. If you can't find unsweetened shredded or flaked coconut at your local market, you can buy it online.

Black and White Beans

Both black and white beans are nutritional powerhouses, chock full of protein, fiber, vitamins, minerals, and antioxidants. I delve into much more about beans and weight loss in chapter 4, but as you start the Rapid Pulse, I'm sure you'll be interested to know that a particular type of fiber in black and white beans, called soluble fiber, has been shown to help reduce belly fat.

This may be due in part to the unique combination of fiber and protein beans contain, a ratio you won't find in any other natural food. Both fiber and protein slow the rate of digestion and absorption, an effect that keeps you fuller longer, delays the return of hunger, and helps regulate blood sugar and insulin levels.

The fiber in black and white beans also has been shown to lower the risk of heart disease and improve digestive health. And like other members of the pulse family, black and white beans help lower the risk of type 2 diabetes, breast and colon cancer, and obesity. The research on pulses is so impressive, it nearly takes my breath away!

What to look for:

Canned black and white beans are absolutely fine—you don't need to soak beans overnight! (I want to make this phase as easy as possible for you.) If possible, look for cans labeled "BPA free" (for more about BPA, see page 270). If you can't find this distinction, look for brands marked "low sodium" or "no added salt." Rinse the beans in a colander under your tap. This step washes away about 40 percent of the sodium.

Sensational Additions

Banana

You may be surprised that a plan designed to kick-start weight loss includes bananas. Yes, they are high in carbohydrates and natural sugar, but bananas aren't "fattening." In fact, they're an amazing choice for both weight loss and health. Bananas are a rich source of potassium, a mineral that acts as a natural diuretic to debloat your body. Potassium also helps maintain calorie-burning muscle mass, and therefore helps keep your metabolism revved.

Banana consumption has also been shown to trigger an increase in dopamine, a neurotransmitter that elevates mood, and whose short supply has been linked to obesity. Bananas are one of the best foods both for sustained energy and a positive mood. The vitamin B_6 in bananas supports mental clarity and an even temperament, and helps regulate blood sugar and insulin levels. This tropical fruit also contains a natural substance called fructooligosaccharides, a prebiotic. Prebiotics are substances that enhance your body's ability to absorb calcium and help "good," probiotic bacteria flourish in your digestive system. More and more studies point to the role of probiotics and healthy gut bacteria in weight control, and consuming more prebiotics is an important step in optimizing your digestive environment.

Finally, bananas provide fiber, and research has shown that every gram of fiber you eat essentially cancels out about 7 calories. This is because fiber bonds to some of the calories you consume and prevents them from being digested and absorbed into your bloodstream, where they have to be either burned or stored. One study found that over six months, each additional gram of fiber dieters consumed resulted in an extra ¼-pound of weight loss.

What to look for:

Bananas are picked from trees while they're still green, and the skins ripen to yellow, then eventually turn black. The best time to eat bananas is when they're firm but not hard, bright yellow, and free from bruises. If you buy all the bananas you need for the Rapid Pulse in one shopping trip, you may want to buy some that are still green or greenish, in addition to some that are yellow. To help protect the planet, I also recommend looking for bananas with a Rainforest Alliance sticker. This signifies that they meet standards that protect ecosystems, wildlife, natural resources, farmers, and farmworkers. Store bananas on the countertop, and if you want to prevent a banana from continuing to ripen, pop it in the fridge. The cold temperature will cause the skin to turn black but will perfectly preserve the fruit.

Tip:

To prevent carb overload, you'll be measuring out your banana portions. Be sure to use a level ½-cup of sliced banana, not a heaping ½-cup!

Figs

Like black beans, figs are a terrific source of filling, weight-loss boosting fiber. They're also loaded with important minerals, including potassium, calcium, and iron. While I haven't found any published research specifically focused on Mission figs, the spectrum of nutrients they contain, their fiber content, and their jet-black hue (and corresponding antioxidants, referenced on page 22) is impressive enough. They also add flavor, texture, and natural sweetness to the Ginger Fig Pulse Pudding.

What to look for:

Find a brand of dried Mission figs that does not contain preservatives, like sulfur dioxide, which can aggravate asthma, allergies, and sensitivities. To avoid preservatives, look for USDA certified organic products or brands that say "unsulfured" or "preservative free." Dried Mission figs don't generally contain added sugar, but read the ingredients list on the package to make sure the only words are "dried figs," "Mission figs," or "black Mission figs."

Your Rapid Pulse Grocery List

Here are all of the ingredients you'll need for the next four days—select the list for the recipe you'll be using.

Ginger Fig Pulse Pudding

- ☑ Bananas, 12 medium (5 to 6 inches long)
- ☑ Chia seeds, 1½ cups (one 12-ounce bag will supply more than you need)
- ☑ Unsweetened coconut milk, 6 cups (two 32-ounce shelf-stable boxes or one refrigerated ½ gallon will supply more than you need)
- ☑ Black beans, four 15.5-ounce cans
- ☑ Figs, one 7-ounce package of dried black Mission figs
- ☑ Fresh ginger, eight 3-inch pieces
- ☑ Unsweetened coconut, ¾ cup or 12 tablespoons (one 7-ounce bag will supply more than you need)

Mango Vanilla Pulse Pudding

☑ Mangos, approximately 6 fresh yellow-skinned

☑ Chia seeds, 1½ cups (one 12-ounce bag will supply more than you
   need)

☑ Unsweetened coconut milk, 6 cups (two 32-ounce, shelf-stable
   boxes or one refrigerated ½ gallon will supply more than you need)

☑ White beans, four 15.5-ounce cans

☑ Vanilla extract (one small bottle of *real* vanilla extract will supply
   more than you need)

☑ Cinnamon (one small jar of ground cinnamon will supply more
   than you need)

☑ Organic honey, 12 tablespoons (optional; one 12-ounce jar will
   supply more than you need)

Dark Chocolate Pulse Pudding

☑ Dates, 36 dried

☑ Chia seeds, 1½ cups (one 12-ounce bag will supply more than you
   need)

☑ Unsweetened coconut milk, 6 cups (two 32-ounce, shelf-stable
   boxes or one refrigerated ½ gallon will supply more than you
   need)

☑ White beans, four 15.5-ounce cans

☑ Vanilla extract (one small bottle of *real* vanilla extract will supply
   more than you need)

☑ Unsweetened cocoa powder, 24 tablespoons (one 8-ounce container
   will supply more than you need)

☑ Organic honey, 12 tablespoons (optional; one 12-ounce jar will
   supply more than you need)

What Can I Drink?

My stance on beverages hasn't changed in years, and I don't think it will, because the science behind it is solid. In a nutshell: though I believe there's a place for tea, as well as a daily coffee treat, the role of beverages is to keep us hydrated, and nothing does that better than plain old H_2O.

Roughly 60 percent of your body is made of water. Water is required for every single bodily process, and even though you don't feel it, every minute of every day you're losing water. Some is lost through normal perspiration, which helps regulate body temperature. You also lose water every time you exhale (you can see it when it's cold outside), and water is needed to create urine, saliva, and other bodily fluids.

The guidelines on water needs from the Institute of Medicine (IOM) haven't changed since I wrote my last book, *S.A.S.S. Yourself Slim*. They state that women aged nineteen and over need 2.7 liters of total fluid per day (over 11 cups) and men need 3.7 liters (over 15 cups). About 20 percent of that water comes from food, which still leaves about 8 to 10 cups each day.

Few people I counsel consistently drink that much. And though I think the payoffs of drinking more water are pretty intuitive, an interesting new study may increase your thirst for water even more. Researchers at the University of Connecticut's Human Performance Laboratory found that even mild dehydration, defined as an approximately 1.5 percent loss in normal fluid volume, can lower your energy level and dampen your mood. The scientists tested healthy women and men who typically worked out thirty to sixty minutes a day. In three separate evaluations, held twenty-eight days apart and at various rates of hydration, each volunteer underwent a battery of tests that measured concentration, reaction time, learning, reasoning, and memory.

Among the women, mild dehydration caused fatigue, headaches, trouble concentrating, and the perception that the tests were more challenging. In the men, mild dehydration compromised memory. The men also experienced fatigue and anxiety while mildly dehydrated, though the mood changes were not as substantial as those experienced by the women. The scientists noted that we don't feel thirsty until we're dehydrated, at which point we're already feeling the effects. The takeaway: if you frequently feel tired, run down, stressed, and brain-foggy, a water shortfall could be a factor.

Though I recommend water above all other beverages, I realize that not everyone—including me—wants to drink nothing but water. So both the Rapid Pulse and the Daily Pulse allow for additional beverages.

Here are the beverages allowed during the Rapid Pulse:

- Water, minimum of 8 cups per day.
- All-natural, calorie-free, flavor-infused flat waters (no bubbles). The only ingredients should be water and natural flavoring, no artificial sweeteners, stevia, or natural sweeteners. (Count this water toward the 8-cup minimum.)
- Fresh, unsweetened brewed iced or hot black, oolong, green, white, red, or herbal tea. Maximum 5 cups per day.
- Bottled unsweetened brewed iced tea. Count toward total tea intake.
- Coffee, limited to 1 cup (8 ounces) per day, with maximum of ¼ cup unsweetened coconut milk. Add 1 teaspoon or one packet of raw sugar, if desired, and flavor with spices, such as cinnamon, nutmeg, or cloves.
- Sweet and Spicy Brew (optional; recipe follows). Count this toward the 5-cup tea maximum.

Sweet and Spicy Brew

1 bag white tea
1½ cups hot water
¼ cup unsweetened coconut milk, warmed
Pinch of ground black cardamom (perhaps 1/32 of a teaspoon)
1 teaspoon blackstrap molasses

Steep the teabag in the hot water for 6 minutes. Pour in the warmed coconut milk, sprinkle in the cardamom, stir in the molasses, and enjoy, sip by sip. For an iced version, chill the brew in the refrigerator overnight and serve it over ice.

Tip: Use your tea brewing time to listen to the five-minute mind massage meditation (see page 46).

This soothing tea, which resembles a chai latte, is delightfully aromatic and, like a latte, can be enjoyed hot or iced. In fact, if you'd like to drink it in place of your daily cup of java, that's perfectly fine. Otherwise, enjoy one portion per day (although this is optional), any time you'd like.

The molasses-cardamom duo, combined with creamy coconut milk, create the sensation of sipping a liquefied gingerbread cookie. And though it's not the prettiest beverage, I think you'll appreciate why I chose each of the ingredients—more black and white benefits. Here's a rundown:

White Tea

White, green, black, and oolong teas all come from the same plant, but they're handled differently. To create black tea, tea leaves are dried and then rolled, a process that cracks the surface of the leaves. Oxygen reacts with enzymes in the leaves, contributing to the characteristic black color. White tea is harvested at a young age, when the buds are covered with fine, silvery hairs—hence the term *white*. Green tea is similar to white, but the leaves are a bit more mature. Oolong tea is in between green and black tea. It tastes richer than green tea but more delicate than black.

There are numerous benefits to drinking tea regularly, including a lower risk of heart disease and stroke, better bone health, protection against age-related memory loss, slower aging, and a reduced risk of type 2 diabetes, breast cancer, glaucoma, and obesity. Though I'm a fan of all tea, white tea, the least processed type, has become my go-to, particularly for weight control.

German researchers conducted a series of experiments on human fat cells and found that exposure to white tea triggered the cells to break down the fat they contain and decreased the expression of genes responsible for the growth of new fat cells.

When researchers from London's Kingston University tested the health properties of twenty-one plant and herb extracts, they found that phenolic-rich white tea outperformed them all. Scientists were specifically looking at each plant's ability to protect the structural proteins elastin and collagen. Elastin supports natural elasticity, which allows lungs, arteries, ligaments, and skin to function properly. It also helps your body's tissues heal when you're injured and stops skin from sagging. Collagen, a protein found in connective tissues, is also important for elasticity as well as cell strength. In the tests, white tea prevented the activities of enzymes that break down elastin and collagen, which can lead to overall aging. The blocked enzymes are also associated with inflammatory diseases, making white tea a powerful combatant of numerous health problems, including type 2 diabetes, rheumatoid arthritis, fibromyalgia, psoriasis, and obesity. Perhaps most significant, the researchers who conducted the study say the amount of white tea responsible for the benefits was quite small, far less than you'd find in a brewed beverage.

Black Cardamom

Black cardamom, a member of the ginger family, is a sweet spice that has been used to treat indigestion, irritable bowel syndrome, constipation, and gas. Cardamom's natural antiflatulence properties make it a wonderful spice to introduce into your diet along with pulses. And because it contains melatonin, a natural hormone released by the body, cardamom also holds promise as a weight-loss secret weapon.

Spanish researchers teamed up with colleagues at the University of Texas Health Science Center in San Antonio to study the effects of melatonin on beige fat, a type of body fat that promotes fat burning. Melatonin is found in small quantities in foods such as mustard, almonds, sunflower seeds, and cherries. The study, conducted in rats, found that melatonin increased the amount of beige fat in both thin and obese animals. Unlike white fat, which gobbles up excess calories and contributes to obesity, beige fat cells are packed with more mitochondria, the tiny furnaces inside cells that burn calories. Carrying just a small amount of this special fat on your frame can result in burning several hundred extra calories a day, which may explain why some people stay slim, seemingly without trying. Right now there's no test to assess how much beige fat you have, but scientists say that exercise is another way to increase levels of beige fat. Research has shown that a hormone called irisin, which is produced during exercise, can trigger white fat cells to produce beige fat.

Note:

Do not use cardamom if you have gallstones or a history of gallstones. In fact, I advise skipping this Sweet and Spicy Brew recipe altogether if you have gallstones, a personal history of gallstones, or a family history of gallstones.

Blackstrap Molasses

Blackstrap molasses starts out as sugarcane, the bamboo-like stalks you may have seen in the produce section of your supermarket. This syrup is a by-product of processing sugarcane into table sugar; essentially, it's the liquid left over after the sugar has crystallized. As a result, it retains concentrated amounts of the nutrients naturally found in sugarcane, including iron, calcium, potassium, magnesium, vitamin B_6, copper, selenium, and manganese. While each of these nutrients is essential, the iron content in blackstrap molasses is particularly beneficial for women, especially those who struggle with low energy. A recent French study looked at the impact of iron on fatigued women and found it to be beneficial, even for those without anemia or low iron stores. In the study, scientists randomly assigned nearly two hundred women ages eighteen to fifty-three to receive either iron or a placebo for twelve weeks. While the blood workups for each of the women showed iron levels in the normal ranges, those who received the mineral had a nearly 50 percent reduction in perceived fatigue, compared to about a 30 percent decline in the placebo group.

Blackstrap molasses is not only full of vitamins and minerals but is also a good source of antioxidants. When Virginia Tech researchers looked at the antioxidant content of several sweeteners, they found that refined sugar, corn syrup, and agave nectar contained minimal antioxidants. Raw

WHY CAN'T I HAVE A SECOND CUP OF JOE?

There are several reasons I chose to limit coffee to 1 cup daily. First, many people can't drink coffee without doctoring it up with extras that can compromise your results. Even if you enjoy your coffee black, it is acidic, so it can irritate your digestive system, something you don't want to do as your body is adjusting to pulses. Also, black coffee has been shown to lower bone density. Finally, in my experience, additional cups of coffee tend to cut into water consumption. If you're going to drink anything besides water, I'd prefer that you reach for tea because of its numerous health benefits. If you're used to drinking lattes, you'll enjoy the Sweet and Spicy Brew, the special creamy drink I introduce in this phase of the plan. It resembles a chai latte, and you can even froth the coconut milk. If you enjoy this beverage, you can continue to drink it for the next thirty days and beyond. After reading about its superstar ingredients, I'm sure you understand why.

cane sugar scored a little higher, followed by maple syrup, brown sugar, and honey, with intermediate antioxidant capacity. But the real standout was blackstrap molasses, which packed the highest antioxidant punch. Though I don't recommend adding sweeteners to meals if you're trying to lose weight, I think the perks of blackstrap molasses make it a worthy inclusion in this one recipe. And a tiny teaspoon goes a long way, offering just enough sweetness bundled with its nutritional benefits.

Can I Exercise During the Rapid Pulse?

Yes, you can work out on my plan, as long as you feel well and energized and as long as you don't engage in strenuous activities, like a spin class or an intense tennis match, or exercise more than an hour a day. The fruits in the pulse puddings—as well as beans—are excellent sources of energy for fueling muscles during workouts. In fact, they're the pre-exercise foods I often recommend to the professional athletes I work with.

Just be sure to time your meals right in relation to the start of your activity. The healthy fat from coconut and the lean protein in the beans slow the rate of digestion and absorption of the good carbs in the pudding. That means you need to give your body a little time to break down the food, so it can be absorbed from your GI tract into your bloodstream. Exercising just after eating the pudding may cause an upset stomach. This is because digestion requires blood to flow to your gut, and when you start exercising, blood flow is diverted to your muscles and cardiovascular system. Though digestion doesn't halt completely, it does slow down. Meanwhile, your meal is trapped in your GI tract, rather than making its way into your blood. This competition for blood flow can cause cramps, poor endurance, and the feeling that there's a brick sitting in your stomach. A good rule of thumb is to wait at least one hour after eating the pudding to start your workout, but no more than ninety minutes. For more info on fitness, please see chapter 8.

QUIT ISN'T IN YOUR VOCABULARY

A few recent surveys revealed some dismal data about dieting. One found that of those who diet regularly, two out of five quit within the first seven days, one out of five last just a month, and the same number—a mere 20 percent—make it to the three-month mark. A second survey found that 37 percent of women say there's no point in starting a diet because they never stick to it for a whole day, let alone a week. The reasons? Nearly 60 percent say they love food too much to diet, and about a quarter point to parties and social events as obstacles. About 20 percent admit to turning to food when they've had a bad day at work.

These are unsettling statistics, to be sure. But I feel confident they won't apply to you. Why? First, because you picked up this book. Even if you don't start this plan right away, just by reading this sentence you've shown you're ready to develop a healthy relationship with food and your body.

Also, many dieters are solely interested in shedding pounds, but because you've chosen to read *this* book, which focuses on both weight loss and optimal health, I bet you are motivated to lose weight and take charge of your personal health simultaneously. That's an incredibly powerful motivator, one that I believe will help you hang in there, even when you feel tempted to settle back into old, unhealthy patterns. In all my years in private practice, and through hearing from women and men around the world who've had success with my previous books, I know that the health transformation you'll experience as a result of adopting this plan will become even more compelling than the pounds and inches you'll lose. To help you connect with that, I'd like you to complete a simple exercise now and every day of this 30-day challenge.

Take out a sheet of paper or grab a sticky note. Close your eyes, take a deep breath, and visualize yourself four days from now, having successfully completed the Rapid Pulse. Picture yourself up to 8 pounds lighter, feeling confident, accomplished, and motivated to transition to the Daily Pulse. Now imagine yourself thirty days from now—not only a full size smaller but also happier, calmer, more well rested, and more energetic.

Scan your body from head to toe. Visualize your shinier hair, glowing skin, healthier heart, stronger digestive system, boosted immunity, and trimmed tummy. Now picture yourself engaging in various activities in this new, slimmer, healthier body, perhaps going for a walk, shopping for new clothes, even dancing alone in your living room. This isn't an imaginary you—this is the you you'll become by staying committed to this plan. Now open your eyes, notice how you feel, and jot down your thoughts. Stash that note in your bag, next to your computer, or someplace handy. When you feel discouraged or inclined to give up, read it and reconnect with that feeling, and that future you. You *can* do this. You *will* become that version of yourself. Just keep going.

. . . .

IS THE SUGAR IN FRUIT BAD?

Absolutely not! None of the top health organizations recommend limiting sugar from whole fruit. The two strictest guidelines on sugar come from the American Heart Association (AHA) and the World Health Organization (WHO), and both focus on added sugar—the sugar you add to coffee or the sugar added by manufacturers to sweeten yogurt, baked goods, cereals, and other processed foods. At this point, nutrition facts labels don't distinguish between naturally occurring sugar (sugar added by Mother Nature) and added sugar (sugar put into the product by the food company), so you have to look beyond the number of sugar grams listed on a package and scrutinize the ingredients list.

For example, if the only ingredient in a bag of dried Mission figs is dried figs, you know that no sugar was added. Because the naturally occurring sugar in fruit is bundled with vitamins, minerals, antioxidants, and fiber, and because it's far less concentrated than added sugars like corn syrup and granulated sugar, it doesn't create the same unwanted effects. In addition, when you eat the Rapid Pulse pudding, the impact of naturally occurring fruit sugar on your blood sugar level is blunted by eating fruit along with lean protein (beans) and good fat (coconut and chia seeds), since both of these macronutrients slow the rate of carbohydrate digestion and absorption. In other words, eating ½ cup of banana slices or fresh mango alone would have a different effect than eating them as part of the pudding.

Is It Okay to Skip the Rapid Pulse?

If you're tempted to skip this phase because you don't think you'll like the pudding, I urge you to try it. Making a fresh start is the perfect time to expand your horizons, get adventurous, and try something new! And if you've been struggling with diet burnout and feeling overwhelmed about losing weight, the break offered by the Rapid Pulse will feel like a blessing. For four days, you won't have to make any decisions about what to eat, when, or how much, because those choices are laid out for you here. You'll only have to prepare food twice. And at the end of those ninety-six hours, you'll have rebooted your metabolism, digestive system, and immune system and resolved an out-of-whack appetite.

That said, if you're feeling hesitant because you've previously rebelled against jump starts, cleanses, detoxes, or limited diets, modifying this phase may be best. For example, if even the thought of being restricted triggers a sense of rebellion that puts you at risk for bingeing, an ultra-limited phase like this may backfire. You know yourself better than anyone, so right now I want you to complete a simple exercise. Take out a sheet of paper. Close your eyes, take a deep breath, ask yourself two questions, then open your eyes and write down exactly what came to you. Here are the questions:

1. When I think about starting the Rapid Pulse, how do I feel emotionally?
2. What does my gut instinct tell me about how my body and mind would respond during this four-day jump start?

Your answers reveal a lot about whether this phase has the potential to be a huge success or a disaster. If your answer to the first question was a positive emotion—excitement, anticipation, hopefulness—the Rapid Pulse may be exactly what you need. But if negative emotions—anxiety, fear, apprehension, doubt—bubbled up, you may wind up begrudging every second of the Rapid Pulse, resenting me, quitting before day four, rebound overeating, and giving up on your goals of losing weight and getting healthy. I don't want any of these things for you. While losing weight is never a walk in the park, I want to make it as easy for you as possible, and I want you to feel well every step of the way.

So if your gut instinct is screaming "Nooooooo!" or "Are you crazy, woman?" modify this phase. Use pudding for one or two of your daily meals, and chose a third meal from the recipes in chapter 5 or the DIY meal-building strategy and lists in chapter 3. You can do the same if you begin the Rapid Pulse and your intuition tells you that it's just not right for you. Remember, this book and plan are about empowering you and giving you tools to make healthy eating and weight loss easier. In my experience, "no pain, no gain" approaches never end well, so there's no place for them in my book.

Beans? Won't I Be Gassy?

I devote chapter 4 entirely to the numerous health and weight-loss benefits of pulses. But even if you're convinced that they deserve a daily place
in your diet, I bet your number one hesitation is their aftereffects, namely
bloating and gas. When I was a kid, I learned the funny song, "Beans,
beans, good for the heart, the more you eat, the more you . . ." Well, you
know the rest. The truth is, if you eat pulses only occasionally, you probably will experience bloating and gassiness, but if you eat them every day,
your body will adjust, and the unwanted side effects will subside. There's
research to support this.

Scientists at Arizona State University tracked forty volunteers for eight
weeks. One group added ½ cup of canned carrots to their diet each day, the
second ½ cup of beans. In the first week, about 35 percent of the subjects
who added beans reported an increase in flatulence; in other words, 65 percent reported no such increase. But by week two, reports of more "tooting"
dropped to 19 percent and continued to decline each week—to 11 percent
for week four and down to 3 percent for week eight. As expected, carrot
eaters, who served as the control group, didn't experience a significant
increase in flatulence, but self-reported bloating was similar between bean
and carrot eaters. During week one, 13 percent of the bean bunch reported
an increase in bloating (so a whopping 87 percent did not); by week eight,
only 2 percent did. Bottom line: though people expect to experience more
gas and bloating from eating beans, reality doesn't match expectations.

If you're still skeptical about how pulses will affect your digestive system, track your symptoms yourself. As the Arizona State study suggests,
you may experience an increase in flatulence within the first week, as your
body adjusts to both the pulses themselves and the boost in your fiber
intake (for more information, see page 209), but it may be far less than you
expect.

For the most accurate assessment, fill out the chart on the next page the
day before you start the Rapid Pulse. Then continue to fill it out daily or

at least weekly (note: this is completely optional!). Passing gas thirteen to twenty-one times a day is considered normal. If you find that you become more flatulent during week one, keep tracking for at least a second week. I anticipate that the flatulence will subside and continue to do so. See page 275 for information about what, besides eating pulses, may trigger gas and bloating, and when to consult your doctor about GI symptoms.

TOOT TRACKER AND BLOAT LOG			
Hour of the day	Each time you toot, make a ✔ or **X** in this column, in the box that corresponds to the hour (for every hour you're awake).	Total number of toots per hour	Make a ✔ or **X** in this column if you feel bloated during the corresponding hour of the day.
5 A.M. hour			
6 A.M. hour			
7 A.M. hour			
8 A.M. hour			
9 A.M. hour			
10 A.M. hour			
11 A.M. hour			
12 P.M. hour			
1 P.M. hour			
2 P.M. hour			
3 P.M. hour			
4 P.M. hour			
5 P.M. hour			
6 P.M. hour			
7 P.M. hour			
8 P.M. hour			
9 P.M. hour			
10 P.M. hour			
11 P.M. hour			
12 A.M. hour			
1 A.M. hour			

Hour of the day	Each time you toot, make a ✔ or **X** in this column, in the box that corresponds to the hour (for every hour you're awake).	Total number of toots per hour	Make a ✔ or **X** in this column if you feel bloated during the corresponding hour of the day.
2 A.M. hour			
3 A.M. hour			
4 A.M. hour			
TOTALS		Total number of toots per day:	Total number of hours per day bloating occurred:

What to Expect During the Rapid Pulse

Your body's reaction to the Rapid Pulse largely depends upon how you were eating before you began this plan. If you were consuming more caffeine and daily doses of foods that contain refined starch (white versions of bread, pasta, rice, crackers) and sugar (candy, sweetened drinks, baked goods), you may experience a *detox* effect. This may include headaches, cravings, and even an anxious feeling for the first day or two, perhaps even into day three. You may also experience a temporary increase in gas and bloating if you were not regularly eating pulses or if your fiber intake was low. Because the three servings of pudding will provide fewer calories than you had been eating, you may also experience hunger, which may be true physical hunger (e.g., stomach rumbling) or simply a desire to eat. The best way to combat this is to either split each pudding into two portions and spread them out a bit, or take your time and really focus on eating slower. Remember that your body has to adjust to eating fewer calories, but the number of calories you were consuming before this plan was *more* than your body needed to get to and stay at a healthy weight. Therefore, a sensation of hunger doesn't mean your body is starving (after all you are giving it fruit, beans, and good fats); it's simply an adjustment period from your former (excessive) norm.

By day three your body should be adjusting nicely, including your digestive system, which is becoming accustomed to the fiber from the fruit, beans, and chia seeds. This trio, along with all the water you're drinking, will have a laxative effect, particularly if you had been experiencing constipation, and that release of built-up waste can be quite a relief! By the end of day three you should feel lighter and more energized, and while I bet you're growing tired of the pudding, your taste buds are being transformed. This transformation will allow you to experience your first Daily Pulse meal with a palate that (after having a break from refined sugar and starch) will appreciate the natural flavors of fresh, whole foods.

By day four you should feel well adjusted to eating on a regular schedule, energized, nourished, and free from headaches or an irritable detox sensation. You should also be more in touch with true sensations of hunger, which may include stomach rumbling within an hour of your scheduled eating times. This is normal and positive, since physical feelings of hunger are something you should be experiencing three times a day. Many people are wary of this at first, but they then learn to embrace it and find that it greatly enhances their enjoyment of meals.

On day four some of the women who tested this plan felt so good they asked if they could stick with the Rapid Pulse for another day or two. Others were more than ready to move on to chewing! The important thing to know is that everyone reacts to a jump start in a unique way, and the best thing you can do is listen to your body. If you do not feel well, or you don't think you can handle eating one more serving of pudding, you always have the option of transitioning to the Daily Pulse at any time, or doing a modified version of this phase. Remember, my goal is for this to be a positive experience, so if for any reason it doesn't feel that way, opt out and start fresh with the Daily Pulse.

The Daily Five-Minute Mind Massage

I am so convinced that meditation can help you lose weight and gain optimal health that I've devoted chapter 7 entirely to this practice. But even before you delve into those pages, I want you to begin experiencing meditation today. Simply log on to my website, www.cynthiasass.com, go to the five-minute mind massage video on the home page, press play, and follow my voice. I've led many people through this exercise, and I promise that after just five minutes, you'll feel significantly more relaxed, refreshed, and renewed. That's why I refer to guided meditation as a "mind massage." During the Rapid Pulse, listen once a day, any time you like, but preferably just before eating one of your puddings. After listening, take a moment to write down your thoughts and reactions in the chart below. In chapter 7, I'll share more about the role these five daily minutes play in supporting weight loss and enhancing your health. For now, just get into the groove of listening once a day and noticing how you feel.

MIND MASSAGE REVELATIONS	
Day	**Mind massage thoughts and reactions** (For example, how did you feel physically and emotionally after listening to the mind massage? What realizations occurred to you?)
1	
2	
3	
4	

NOT ALL WHITE FOODS ARE CREATED EQUAL

As I've demonstrated in this chapter, some of the healthiest foods on the planet are pasty pale. In addition to bananas, coconut, white beans, and ginger, other wonderful white foods include garlic, onions, pears, mushrooms, cauliflower, jicama, and potatoes, as well as white versions of asparagus, eggplant, nectarines, peaches, corn, and parsnips. You'll find these referenced in chapter 3. Some white foods, however, do deserve to be shunned. Processed white foods, like white flour and sugar, are stripped of their nutrients, wreak havoc with blood sugar and insulin regulation, and are tied to both obesity and type 2 diabetes. You won't find them in this plan.

However, in all my years of counseling clients, I know it's not realistic to go through life eating perfectly 100 percent of the time. So, if you feel the need to indulge, you'll find healthy versions of treats in chapter 6, including brownies and mini pumpkin muffins. None of these recipes contain white sugar or flour, and I bet you'll find them just as satisfying, if not more so, than their traditionally made counterparts. And if, for whatever reason, you do eat something that includes the "bad whites," I've included advice about how to undo the damage and get back on track starting on page 301.

WHY THE SPOON YOU CHOOSE MATTERS

In a 2013 study, published in the journal *Flavour,* scientists found that yogurt was perceived as denser and more expensive when it was tasted from a light plastic spoon, compared to a heavier, metal spoon. While I'm not a fan of plastic anything, this trick may be helpful during the Rapid Pulse, particularly due to the research tying a thicker consistency to a boost in fullness.

IS IT OKAY TO FOLLOW THE RAPID PULSE IF I HAVE DIABETES?

No. This plan is designed for healthy adults with no chronic illnesses or conditions that require a special or therapeutic diet. Anyone with diabetes or any other chronic condition should skip the Rapid Pulse. The Daily Pulse plan is very much in line with the current diabetes management guidelines, but it's always important to check with your doctor and get his or her approval before changing your diet or beginning a new eating plan.

HOW TO COPE WHEN YOU CRAVE OTHER FOODS

Do you worry that eating pudding three times a day will cause you to crave other splurge foods? Here's a trick to stave off cravings: choose an image that's meaningful to you and visualize it when you're feeling tempted by cravings. Or keep a small bottle of eucalyptus oil on hand and sniff it to break a craving.

As a recent Australian study found, this strategy works! Volunteers who craved chocolate were so distracted by their cravings they took longer to solve math problems and they weren't able to recall as much information. But when the same volunteers were asked to envision a nonfood image, like a rainbow, or to recall nonfood smells, such as eucalyptus, their cravings subsided. The researchers found that the strength of cravings is linked to how vividly people imagine a food, so do what you can to avoid creating a vibrant picture of other foods in your mind.

My Story

Joy Bennett, age 39

Lost 18 pounds and 16.5 inches

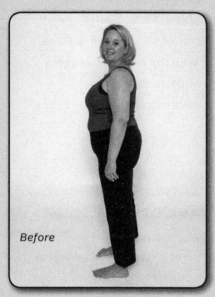

Before

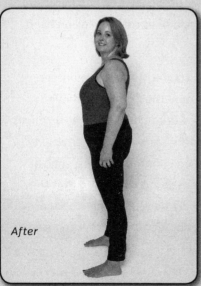

After

Before this plan my eating was actually pretty healthy, but I did eat a couple of fast food meals per week. I also never ate breakfast and would often go many, many hours between meals.

What surprised me most about this experience was that this plan is really easy! I didn't think it would be so simple to follow and stay on track. I really like the wardrobe explanation of how to construct my meals. It made it very simple and straightforward for me. I also really liked not having to follow a recipe in order to get all the requirements in one meal. I quickly became comfortable with the wardrobe design and confident about throwing a meal together and staying within the guidelines.

My favorite meals were the Black Bean "Tacos," the Basil Balsamic Tuna Salad, and the Garlicky Shrimp Scampi. Real food—and within two weeks I was wearing shorts that hadn't fit me for over two years!!!!

20 21 22 23 24 25 26 27 28 29 30 31 32 33 34 35 36 3

••

This 30-day challenge taught me that I can feel good without caffeine and junk food. I also learned how much more energy I had by eating breakfast and that I didn't need to snack. I didn't need the junk I was eating! The other thing I have noticed is this is not an expensive way to eat. I will admit at first I was concerned that this would make me go over my budget, but it hasn't.

I plan to continue this plan, maybe allowing myself a few days a month off, but I really liked how easy this is and how I feel when I eat this way. My skin is much better, and I look healthier. Overall I'm also in better moods and have much more energy. It's been great!

[3]

The Daily Pulse

Congratulations! You made it through the Rapid Pulse! I know you probably don't want to hear the word *pudding* for a while, but you did it! In just ninety-six hours, you've made a giant leap forward, not only in your weight-loss journey but also in transforming your physical and emotional well-being. You've started to come alive again, reconnect with your appetite, and learn to trust your body's built-in mechanisms for guiding you back into balance.

Now it's time to take advantage of that momentum and keep moving forward, using phase two, the Daily Pulse. By the end of this chapter, you'll have mastered a simple meal-building method—one that will allow you to continue shedding pounds and inches for the next twenty-six days while enjoying a much broader array of delicious, nutrient-rich meals. (Hello, Basil Balsamic Tuna Salad and Broccoli Cashew Chicken Stir-Fry—two of the testers' favorite recipes from chapter 5!)

If you're not yet ready to learn the "whys" of this phase and you just want to "keep doing," you can skip to chapter 5 now, follow my simple instructions, choose recipes you like, and prepare them as described. But when you're ready, I want you to understand the framework behind those recipes. That's what this chapter is all about.

Once you grasp the strategy laid out in the next several pages, you'll have a simple, savvy tactic for creating your own meals, ordering from restaurant menus, or modifying any recipe to fall in line with your new weight-loss plan. In fact, once I teach you my crafty approach for assembling your three daily meals, you'll be able to walk through the grocery aisles and know exactly what to put into your cart, or open your fridge or cupboards and know precisely what and how much to include in a meal and why. This knowledge will unburden you from the uncertainty and confusion most people struggle with when trying to lose weight. This chapter will also give you the freedom and confidence to make the best choices under any given circumstances, develop a consistent, slimming eating pattern, and allow you to achieve real and lasting results—all while feeling healthy and energized. Are you ready to dive in?

The Wardrobe Analogy

In my work, I do a lot of explaining. I want my clients to understand the reasoning behind my philosophies, and over the years I have found that nothing helps make a concept more clear than an analogy. When you can connect a science-based concept to an aspect of your day-to-day life, the concept instantly becomes understandable, and acting on it makes perfect sense. My analogy for this phase of the plan is simple: think of each meal as an outfit, put together with three basic wardrobe staples plus an accessory. It couldn't get much easier.

And this is why the analogy is so fitting (pardon the pun!). One day, when talking to a fashion-forward client, I used a wardrobe analogy, and it connected for her in a way that suddenly made everything crystal clear. She was lamenting that she had no idea how to put healthy meals together that would allow her to lose weight, and she was confused about what to eat. I said, "Well, it's kind of like putting together an outfit. You wouldn't walk out the door wearing two pairs of pants and no top, right? In the same way, you shouldn't double up on carbs and skip the protein, or vice versa." When my client heard this, her body language softened, her eyes lit up, and she said, "Nobody ever explained it to me like that before—I get it!" When other clients also responded with lightbulb moments, I knew I had stumbled upon a concept that would form the structure of this eating plan. Here's how it works.

Rule #1:
Build Your Meals Using the Wardrobe Design

Each of your three daily meals will include three diet wardrobe staples: lean protein plus veggies plus plant-based fat. Think a top, a bottom, and footwear—three must-have elements.

At each meal, you'll also add one of four possible accessories, which I'm calling your *energy accessory:*

Whole grain

or

Starchy vegetable

or

Fruit

or

Pulse

You also have the option of adding a half serving of two of these accessories.

The possibilities are endless. Lean protein plus veggies plus plant-based fat could be as diverse as grilled chicken breast plus broccoli florets plus olive oil (seasoned with garlic and herbs), or scrambled eggs plus onions, tomato, and spinach plus sliced avocado (flavored with cilantro). You'll find an array of delicious and well-matched choices in chapter 5. Your energy accessory options are similarly wide ranging. Oven-roasted sweet potatoes, chilled lentils, a cup of fresh strawberries, and popped popcorn are all fair game.

Rule #2:
Include a Pulse Serving in at Least One Daily Meal

Another critical rule in this phase is that at least ONE of your meals must include a pulse, the superstar of this plan, and you have two options for doing this:

- Choose a pulse as the energy accessory (the *plus-pulse* option)

or

- Choose a meal with a pulse as the lean protein (the *pulse-as-protein* option)

I introduced you to the power of pulses in chapter 1, and as I'm sure you've already gathered, consuming at least one daily pulse serving is an important part of how this plan works, both for weight loss and to optimize your health. That's why I call this phase the Daily Pulse.

In terms of how pulses fit into a meal, they are unique because they serve double duty. They are a plant-based lean protein, so you'll find them listed in the protein section on page 67. The recipes in chapter 5 are arranged based on their protein source, so to choose a *pulse-as-protein* meal, flip to the pulse section on page 82. In addition, because pulses also contain complex carbohydrates, they can likewise be categorized in this plan as an accessory, specifically an energy accessory.

Energy accessories are foods that fuel your body's cells, allowing them to perform their vital functions, much like gasoline in your car. When you choose a meal with pulse as the energy accessory, the *plus-pulse* option, you'll also get a bit of bonus protein. Many of the testers reported that these plus-pulse meals were their favorites. The pulses' dynamic duo of protein and carbohydrate left them feeling both satisfied and energized, unlike previous low-carb diet attempts, which left them feeling fatigued and craving carbs.

So, to recap, each of your three daily meals will include the following:

Lean protein

Veggies

Plant-based fat

+ Energy accessory (whole grain *or* **starchy vegetable** *or* **fruit** *or* **pulse** *or* **half servings of two of these)**

In at least one of your daily meals, you must include a pulse. Because pulses serve double duty, your two pulse meal options are

Plus-Pulse Option:

Lean protein

Veggies

Plant-based fat

+ Pulse as the energy accessory

or

Pulse-as-Protein Option:

Pulse as your lean protein

Veggies

Plant-based fat

+ Energy accessory

Are you thinking, *Wait, what counts as plant-based fat?* or *Are carrots a starchy vegetable?* or *How much fruit can I eat?* Just hang on! In this chapter, I list every food that counts within each of these categories, in addition to the serving sizes allowed. I've also included illustrations and a handy cheat sheet to help you memorize the wardrobe design, so you can train your brain to think about putting meals together in this way. Plus, every meal in chapter 5 is a "complete outfit," so by simply studying the meals and preparing the recipes, you'll find that this meal-building strategy will quickly become second nature.

Rule #3:
You Don't Need to Clean Your Plate

Try to slow down when eating, listen to your body, and stop when full, even if you haven't finished your meal. You may find that the exact same meal feels like a perfect amount one day and a bit too much another. That's completely normal, since your hunger/fullness patterns can be influenced by a number of factors, including your activity level, hormonal shifts, even the weather. If you ever feel like a full meal isn't enough, be sure to revisit the Two Additional Accessory Rules on page 90 to learn how to add. But when a meal feels like more than your body needs at the moment, honor your fullness signals and stop when you hit the just-right amount.

Rule #4:
Time Your Meals Right

As you did during the Rapid Pulse, eat your first meal within an hour of waking. Eat your second meal four to five hours later, and eat your third meal four to five hours after that. For example

Meal 1—9 A.M.
Meal 2—1 P.M.
Meal 3—6 P.M.

or

Meal 1—8 A.M.
Meal 2—12 P.M.
Meal 3—5 P.M.

or

Meal 1—7 A.M.
Meal 2—12 P.M.
Meal 3—5 P.M.

You may have noticed that I refer to three meals a day, rather than specifying breakfast, lunch, and dinner. That's because all of the meals in this phase, including those in chapter 5, have the same structure and are therefore interchangeable. I've chosen this approach because many of my clients enjoy eating traditional lunch or dinner foods, like a casserole, for breakfast, or they prefer to eat an omelet or quiche for dinner, and that's perfectly okay. So in chapter 5, instead of seeing the meals listed as breakfast, lunch, and dinner options, you'll see them listed according to their protein source—eggs, dairy, poultry, seafood, or pulse. You can enjoy any of these meals as meal 1, 2, or 3, or use the meal-building strategy in this chapter to craft your own.

If you're not used to eating veggies at breakfast, remember that just 4 ounces (½ cup) of 100 percent vegetable juice counts, which you can either purchase premade or juice yourself and gulp down before you begin prepping the rest of your meal. You can also opt to whip veggies into a fruit smoothie, as I have in the recipes on pages 124 and 132, or you can start or end your first meal with a crisp side of raw veggies. For example, some of the women who tested this plan enjoyed nibbling on a cup of sliced bell peppers and cucumbers, either as they made their oatmeal or parfait, or as a palate cleanser afterward. Others fell in love with starting each day with a veggie omelet, or enjoying "dinner for breakfast" and opting for a savory meal, like Chilled Pesto Cheesy Salad or Lemon Pepper Hummus.

SHOULD YOU FAST FOR SIXTEEN HOURS EACH DAY?

Actor Hugh Jackman has publicly shared that he got in shape for his *X-Men* role in part by limiting his food intake to eight hours a day and fasting for the remaining sixteen. Dubbed "the Wolverine diet," this intermittent fasting approach has attracted other celebs, including Viola Davis. It became popular after a rat study was published in the journal *Cell Metabolism*. Scientists put three groups of rodents on different diets for one hundred days. One group was fed healthy fare, while the other two groups chowed on fattening feed. Half of the junk food eaters were allowed to eat whenever they wanted to. The others had access to food only for the eight hours they were most active. Researchers found that the rats that ate a fatty diet but were forced to fast for sixteen hours were almost as lean as those who ate the healthy fare. While this is certainly interesting, I think it's pretty darn tough for humans to pull off.

If you wake up at 7 A.M. and eat breakfast within an hour, you'd have to eat your third meal no later than about 4 P.M. Technically, that could fit my meal timing rules—for example, if you ate meal 1 at 7:30 A.M., meal 2 at 11:30 A.M. and meal 3 at 3:30 P.M. But if you get eight hours of sleep, that would mean a seven-and-a-half-hour stretch between your last meal and hitting the hay. I tried this myself, and I just couldn't do it. My grumbling tummy made it difficult to fall asleep, and ultimately, I had to get up and eat some nuts. If you want to experiment for yourself, give it a try, but keep in mind that my goal for you isn't just weight loss. It's also optimal health, which includes both physical and emotional well-being. For this, you need to adopt a sane, sensible plan you can stick with long term. If you find that nighttime fasting makes you cranky, interferes with your sleep, triggers intense hunger or cravings, or makes you want to throw in the towel and give up on losing weight completely, ditch this approach and spread out your meals a bit more. For example, eating meal 1 at 8 A.M., meal 2 at 1 P.M., and meal 3 at 6 P.M. may make all the difference in helping you hang in there and feel happy.

DIET WARDROBE STAPLES

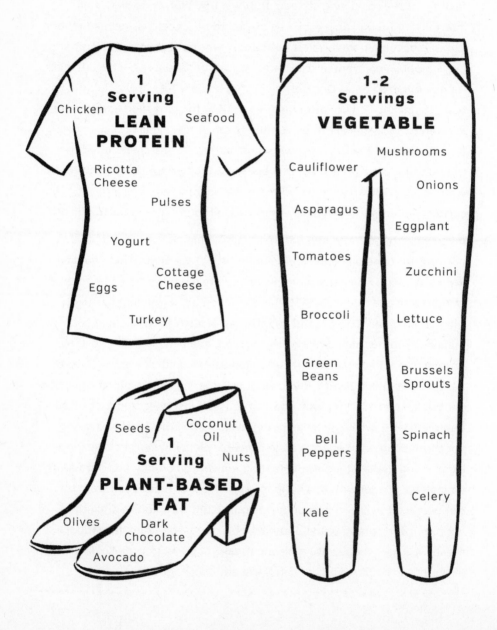

1
Serving
LEAN PROTEIN

Chicken
Seafood
Ricotta Cheese
Pulses
Yogurt
Cottage Cheese
Eggs
Turkey

1-2
Servings
VEGETABLE

Cauliflower
Mushrooms
Onions
Asparagus
Eggplant
Tomatoes
Zucchini
Broccoli
Lettuce
Green Beans
Brussels Sprouts
Bell Peppers
Spinach
Kale
Celery

1
Serving
PLANT-BASED FAT

Seeds
Coconut Oil
Nuts
Olives
Dark Chocolate
Avocado

ENERGY ACCESSORIES
Choose
1 or 1/2 portions
from 2

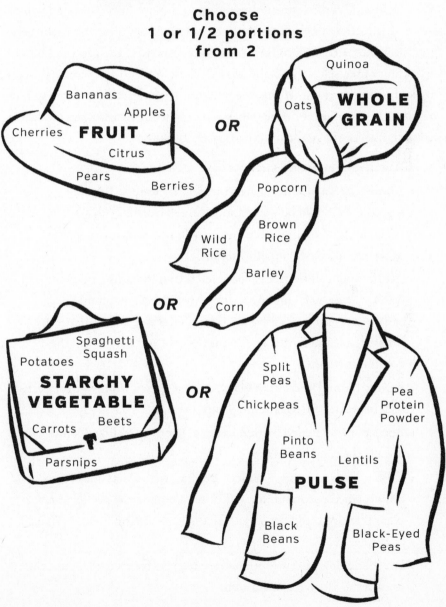

FRUIT

Bananas
Apples
Cherries
Citrus
Pears
Berries

OR

WHOLE GRAIN

Quinoa
Oats
Popcorn
Brown Rice
Wild Rice
Barley
Corn

OR

STARCHY VEGETABLE

Spaghetti Squash
Potatoes
Carrots
Beets
Parsnips

OR

PULSE

Split Peas
Chickpeas
Pea Protein Powder
Pinto Beans
Lentils
Black Beans
Black-Eyed Peas

Rule #5: Drink Only the Approved Beverages

In this phase, you'll enjoy the same beverage options as during the Rapid Pulse, with the addition of carbonated waters. During the kick start, as your body adjusted to consuming pulses and more fiber, I wanted you to avoid drinks that might contribute to bloating. I'm allowing them here, but please pay attention to how your body responds. The gassy bubbles in sparkling water, seltzer, or club soda can cause your GI tract to swell like a balloon filling with air. If this becomes bothersome, stick to flat water, or reserve fizzy versions for times when bloating won't be a bother, like when you're home for the night and wearing comfy clothes.

- Water, minimum of 8 cups per day
- All-natural, calorie-free, flavor-infused flat waters. The only ingredients should be water and natural flavoring—no artificial sweeteners, no natural sweeteners, including stevia. Count this water toward the 8-cup minimum.
- All-natural, calorie-free carbonated water, including sparkling water, seltzer, and club soda. The only ingredients should be carbonated water or carbonated mineral water and, if flavor infused, natural flavoring. Count these beverages toward the 8-cup minimum.
- Freshly brewed iced or hot black, oolong, green, white, red, or herbal tea, unsweetened. Maximum 5 cups per day.
- Bottled unsweetened brewed iced tea, flat or sparkling. Count toward the total tea intake.
- Coffee, limit to 1 cup (8 ounces) per day, with a maximum of ¼ cup unsweetened coconut milk. Add 1 teaspoon or one packet of raw sugar if desired, and flavor with spices, such as cinnamon, nutmeg, or cloves.
- Sweet and Spicy Brew (optional; see page 33 for recipe). Count this toward the 5-cup tea maximum.

FACT The average American consumes 78 pounds of sweeteners per person per year, mostly from sugar and high-fructose corn syrup. That's the equivalent of 8,853 teaspoons annually, more than 1¼ cups per person each and every day!

Why Energy Accessories?

The terms *carbohydrate, carbs,* and *starch* have negative connotations these days. Many weight-loss plans cut them out altogether, and while that may be a simple approach, it isn't optimal or practical. Even my clients who experienced significant weight loss on low-carb diets ultimately abandoned them due to bothersome side effects, including irritability, mood swings, fatigue, headaches, low blood sugar, digestive upset, constipation, and constant cravings. They describe experiencing "carb withdrawal" or feeling "zombie-like."

Because low-carb diets have become incredibly popular, I tested this approach myself, and I thought my husband was going to divorce me! My normally calm demeanor was replaced with chronic edginess. Every little thing got on my nerves. I had trouble concentrating, lacked the energy to exercise, and had difficulty falling asleep and staying asleep, and my digestive system was very unhappy (I'll spare you the details!). Plus, I constantly daydreamed about potatoes, fruit, and pulses! Yes, I could have guacamole, but only without black beans. Almond butter was okay, but I couldn't enjoy it swirled into oatmeal or spread onto tart apple slices. And as much as I love vegetables, I was downright miserable without my usual favorite foods, like grapes, popcorn, potatoes, and lentils. I also felt awful about missing out on the abundance of nutrients I know those foods are chock full of. I felt like I was robbing my body of nutrition and short-changing my health. This experience solidified my viewpoint on low-carb diets: even if you lose weight, eliminating carbs is no way to live, and it's certainly not the right way to achieve optimal health. Avoiding carbs is also not necessary in order to lose weight!

Carbs aren't inherently evil. Though there are some high-carb foods I want you to avoid, like refined grains and sugar, the approach that makes the most sense for both weight loss and health is to include the right type of starchy foods, in the right amounts, at the right times. Rather than cutting out carbs altogether, I've put them into their proper place in each meal and described them as what they really are: energy accessories.

Here's the deal about carbs: Their only role in your diet is to fuel active cells. Nothing in your body is made out of carbohydrate, so starchy foods don't provide raw materials for maintaining, healing, or repairing your body's tissues. In a nutshell, when you digest and absorb carbohydrate, and it makes its way to your cells, one of four things will happen to it, in the following order:

First, your cells will burn the available carb for fuel—if they need it.

Second, if the cells don't need the fuel at that moment, either because they already have enough or because your energy demand is low (for example, you're on the couch watching TV), the unneeded carb energy will get converted into a substance called glycogen, the storage form of carbohydrate. Glycogen is like a starch piggy bank your body can rely on if needed. You store some glycogen in your liver; it's used to keep your blood sugar level steady as you sleep and replenish blood sugar if it dips too low. You also store quite a bit of glycogen in your muscle tissue, where it is used to provide an immediate fuel source to muscle cells when they're active, such as during a long walk, a climb up some stairs, or a fast-paced bike ride.

Third, if your glycogen piggy banks are full, your body sends surplus carbohydrate to your fat cells, where the carbs feed the fat you already have, thus maintaining it.

Fourth, if your fat cells are adequately fed, your body converts the excess carbs into new fat and socks it away in your fat cells, plumping them up even more.

One of the reasons I'm explaining all of this is because I want you to know it's not true that carbs are intrinsically fattening. Of the four possible fates of carbohydrate—(1) burned off as fuel; (2) stored as glycogen; (3) used to feed and maintain current fat tissue; or (4) converted into new fat—the first two are pretty darned important. That's why I want you to include some type of healthy starch in each meal. But to prevent winding up with an excess of carbs, which would lead to fates 3 and 4, you're only going to include starchy foods as accessories. Bottom line: the right type of carbohydrate-rich foods in the right amounts (which are laid out in this chapter as well as in the recipes in chapter 5) at the right times (see page 59) will allow you to enjoy the energy and nutrients these foods provide while successfully starving the fat tissue you don't want to keep.

THE CARB MISTAKE HEALTHY PEOPLE MAKE

One of the biggest barriers to weight loss I've witnessed in my private practice is healthy overaccessorizing. I've seen many people switch from refined grains to whole grains, thinking that healthier eating—for example, eating quinoa with dinner instead of white rice—will trigger weight loss. But healthy foods aren't innately slimming. Any time you take in more carbohydrate, even from nutrient-rich sources, than your body needs to support your ideal weight, the surplus will prevent you from seeing results. In these cases, the solution isn't to ditch carb-rich foods like quinoa completely, but instead to cut back to amounts that ensure all the carbohydrate you consume will be burned off or converted into glycogen and burned later. I can't say it enough: getting carbs right is all about choosing the right type of carbs in the right amounts and at the right times.

Okay, now that we've talked through the wardrobe design, let's explore your three diet wardrobe staples (lean protein plus veggies plus plant-based fat) and your accessory options (whole grain *or* starchy vegetable *or* fruit *or* pulse) in more detail.

Instead of, or in addition to, relying on the recipes in chapter 5, you can use the lists and corresponding portions on the next pages of this chapter to craft your own meals using the wardrobe design.

Each meal should include

- 1 serving of lean protein
- 1 or 2 servings of veggies (your choice, or include 1½ servings)
- 1 serving of plant-based fat
- 1 serving of an energy accessory, or half portions of two of these options (choose from whole grain *or* starchy vegetable *or* fruit *or* pulse)

For example

- Lean protein: 3 ounces of grilled chicken breast
- Veggies: 2 cups of roasted eggplant, bell peppers, cauliflower, and tomatoes
- Plant-based fat: 1 tablespoon of extra-virgin olive oil (half on the veggies, half on the potatoes)
- Energy accessory (starchy vegetable option): ½ cup of roasted red potatoes

Also, you need to make sure that one of your daily meals includes a pulse, either a plus-pulse meal, with pulse as the energy accessory, or a pulse-as-protein meal, with pulse as the lean protein. For example

Plus-pulse meal: Southwest omelet
- Lean protein: 1 whole organic egg and 3 whites
- Veggies: 2 cups chopped tomatoes, mushrooms, onions, and spinach
- Plant-based fat: ¼ of a ripe avocado, sliced
- Energy accessory: ½ cup cooked black beans

Pulse-as-protein meal: chilled lentil and quinoa salad
- Lean protein: ½ cup cooked, chilled lentils
- Veggies: 2 cups baby spinach leaves

- Plant-based fat: 2 tablespoons tahini (to dress the spinach)
- Energy accessory (whole-grain option): ½ cup cooked, chilled quinoa

Diet Wardrobe Staple: Lean Protein

Protein is part of every cell in your body, including your muscles, organs, skin, hair, red blood cells, hormones, and immune cells. The chief role of protein in your diet is to maintain, heal, repair, and build tissues in your body. In essence, your body is like one magnificent, perpetual construction site. Each and every day you use protein to replace cells that have died off, repair those that have become damaged, and build tissues that rely on protein for their structure. If you take in too little protein, many of these jobs can't get done, and before long, you'll see and feel the effects. A protein shortfall can trigger the loss of muscle mass, a weaker immune system, dry skin, dull hair or hair loss, and hormone imbalances.

On the flip side, too much protein can also cause unwanted side effects. When your body has more protein than it needs for all of its construction work, the surplus can contribute to weight gain or prevent weight loss. In other words, if there are no cells that need to be built, maintained, or repaired, your body will have raw materials it cannot use. When this is the case, your body has no choice but to shuttle surplus protein to your fat cells. Many people are shocked to learn that the reason they're carrying a spare tire or muffin top is that they're taking in too much protein. But again, it's like a construction site. If too much steel is delivered to a site, more than a project calls for, builders won't just tack it onto the structure without purpose; it piles up as surplus.

To help you achieve the best balance, I include one serving of lean protein in every meal. The list of lean protein options includes pulses, as well as animal-based foods, but there are a few you won't find on the list. To learn why I left off red meat, milk, hard cheeses, and soy, see pages 69–71.

In addition to helping build and repair body tissues, protein helps regulate blood sugar and insulin levels, and keeps you fuller longer by slowing the rate of digestion and absorption. If you've ever eaten a low-protein, high-carb meal, such as a bowl of pasta with tomato sauce, you've probably noticed how quickly you're hungry again.

One serving of lean protein equals

- ½ cup cooked pulses (beans, peas, lentils—see the full list below)
- ¼ cup unsweetened pea protein powder
- 6 ounces nonfat organic yogurt, preferably Greek
- ½ cup organic egg whites or 1 whole organic egg and 3 whites
- ½ cup organic nonfat cottage cheese
- ¼ cup organic nonfat ricotta cheese
- 3 ounces poultry or seafood

Pulse proteins include

- Beans: all varieties, including adzuki, anasazi, black, cranberry, cannellini, Dutch brown, fava, flageolet, great northern, kidney, lima, marrow, mung, navy, pigeon, pink, pinto, and red
- Peas: black-eyed peas, chickpeas (garbanzo beans), split peas, green peas, and unsweetened pea protein powder
- Lentils: all varieties, including brown, black, green, red, and yellow

Animal-based proteins include

- Organic eggs
- Nonfat organic cottage cheese
- Nonfat organic ricotta cheese
- Nonfat organic yogurt
- Chicken: boneless skinless breast and at least 93 percent lean ground chicken
- Turkey: boneless skinless breast and at least 93 percent lean ground turkey
- Seafood

WHERE DOES HUMMUS COUNT?

Hummus is typically made from chickpeas and either tahini (sesame seed paste) or olive oil or both, along with seasonings like lemon juice and garlic. So ¼ cup of hummus would count as both the lean protein (pulse) and the plant-based fat in a meal. If you'd like to make it yourself, see my recipe on page 160. And for on-the-go meals that include store-bought hummus, flip to page 272.

WHY ISN'T RED MEAT ON THE LIST?

Americans consume 74 pounds of red meat per person annually—that's the equivalent of more than one smartphone-size portion per person every day of the year, and all that red meat may be contributing to America's diabetes epidemic. A 2013 study, based on Harvard data and published in *JAMA Internal Medicine,* found that men and women who increased their red meat consumption by more than half a serving per day over four years increased their risk of developing diabetes over the ensuing four years by 48 percent. By contrast, those who reduced their red meat consumption by more than a half serving per day lowered their risk of developing diabetes by 14 percent.

Another recent Harvard study found that women who averaged two servings of red meat daily had a 30 percent higher risk of developing heart disease than women who averaged half a serving per day. The scientists also found that replacing red meat with other lean proteins helped lower heart disease risk. Compared to women who ate one daily serving of red meat, women who ate fish had a 24 percent lower heart disease risk. Those who ate poultry instead of red meat had a 19 percent lower risk of developing heart disease, and those who ate low-fat dairy products instead of a daily red meat serving lowered their heart disease risk by 13 percent. Additionally, over a twenty-eight-year period, women who consumed an average of one daily serving of unprocessed red meat, such as a piece of steak, had a 13 percent increased risk of early death, and those who averaged one daily serving of processed red meat, such as a hot dog or two slices of bacon, had a 20 percent greater chance of dying.

Yet another study found that inflammation resulting from the consumption of red meat may spur cancer by promoting tumor cell growth. These are just a handful of the studies that have linked red meat to health risks. The research is so compelling that I chose not to make red meat a daily option. However, if you don't want to cut out red meat completely, build it in as an occasional splurge. See page 301 for how.

WHY NO MILK AND HARD CHEESE?

Over the years, I've noticed that among my clients, those who consume hard cheese and milk often don't lose as much weight as those who forego these dairy products or eat them only occasionally. I believe this is because even if the portions are controlled, a serving of hard cheese provides less protein and far more animal-based fat than 3 ounces of poultry or seafood. In addition, a cup of milk packs nearly twice as much carbohydrate as protein, without the beneficial fiber and antioxidants found in pulses. For these reasons, the only dairy products I've chosen to include in my plan are nonfat and high in protein. However, if, like my husband, Jack, you can't live without hard cheese or if you sometimes crave a glass of milk, you can enjoy them as occasional splurges. To learn how, see page 301.

FACT In 1980, Americans consumed about 8 pounds of cheese per person per year. Today we're gobbling 23 pounds per person per year. That's equivalent to 368 slices each annually! To work off all that gooey dairy, you'd have to walk swiftly for four and a half days straight.

WHAT IF I CAN'T LIVE WITHOUT CHEESE (OR MILK OR RED MEAT . . .)?

I don't want you to give up before you get started. So if you don't think you can give up steak, cheese, or any other food not built into the daily framework of this plan, turn to How to Squeeze In a Splurge on page 301. There, you'll learn how to include any can't-live-without food without compromising your results.

NO SOY ALLOWED?

In my previous two weight-loss books, I included soy as a lean protein option, but not this time. Like many people I've talked to over the past few years, I personally developed a severe soy intolerance. My experience, which I describe in more detail starting on page 265, led me to rethink my stance on soy and omit it as a recommended option. However, if you love tofu or edamame and don't want to give it up, see page 266 for how to swap it in.

CHOOSE SUSTAINABLE SEAFOOD

Seafood is a bit of a nutritional catch-22: it's loaded with healthy omega-3s but may contain harmful levels of mercury. To help consumers sort out how to reap the benefits without incurring the risks, the Monterey Bay Aquarium's Seafood Watch program created an important guide. On your computer or smartphone, log on to www.seafoodwatch .org or download the free app. On the site or within the app you'll find the Super Green list. Updated regularly, this list includes only the fish that meet three key criteria: each is (1) environmentally sustainable (so we'll still have fresh seafood for years to come); (2) low in mercury; and (3) high in healthful omega-3s. I strongly encourage you to use this resource. For more info on mercury, including a calculator that estimates your exposure, visit the Natural Resources Defense Council site at www .nrdc.org/health/effects/mercury/guide.asp.

Diet Wardrobe Staple: Veggies

From a botany perspective, anything that doesn't qualify as a fruit (produce that forms from plant flowers and contains seeds) is considered a vegetable. However, my definition of a vegetable is more practical than technical. Foods we think of as fruits are sweet, and those we consider vegetables are less sweet. So while tomatoes and cucumbers are fruits, botanically speaking, I've listed them here as veggies.

I've chosen veggies as a diet wardrobe staple because in addition to being low in calories and loaded with water and fiber, veggies are packed with nutrients most of us fall short on each day, including potassium, magnesium, folate, and vitamins A, C, and K. Plus, a higher intake of veggies is tied to a lower risk of several chronic diseases, including obesity, as well as heart disease and cancer, the top two killers in America.

According to the latest data, just 26.3 percent of Americans eat three daily servings of vegetables, the minimum recommended. In this plan, I include one to two veggie servings in every meal (see page 108 for the meal framework), so you'll easily rack up at least three a day.

 Some vegetables contain as much carbohydrate as whole grains and fruits, which makes them more appropriate as energy accessory options than meal staples. You'll find this list on page 79.

One vegetable serving equals

- 1 cup fresh or frozen veggies (measured from frozen state)
- ¼ cup preservative-free dried veggies, such as sundried tomatoes
- 4 ounces (½ cup) of 100 percent vegetable juice (purchased or juiced at home)

Vegetables include

Artichokes	Green beans
Arugula	Kale
Asparagus	Lettuce (all varieties)
Bell peppers	Mushrooms
Bok choy	Okra
Broccoli	Onions
Broccoli rabe	Peppers
Broccolini	Radicchio
Brussels sprouts	Radishes
Cabbage	Snow peas
Cauliflower	Spinach
Celery	Sugar snap peas
Collard greens	Swiss chard
Cucumbers	Tomatoes (all varieties)
Eggplant	Watercress
Endive	Yellow wax beans
Fennel	Zucchini

While green beans and yellow wax beans are in the same family as other beans, they aren't considered pulses because they're picked while still immature, just as the beans are beginning to form, and are consumed pod and all.

Diet Wardrobe Staple: Plant-Based Fat

Fat is one of the most important nutrients in your diet. Fats are a structural part of your cells, which means you can't heal cells or construct new ones without this key building block. Fats are also needed to maintain healthy skin and hair, and they're necessary for absorbing certain antioxidants and the fat-soluble vitamins. These vitamins, A, D, E, and K, grab on to fat as they are transported from your digestive system into your blood. According to the Institute of Medicine, fat should make up an even higher percentage of your total calorie intake than protein. For these reasons, fat is an essential meal component, but not all fats have equal effects on health. In this plan, I focus on plant-based fats, which in addition to being heart-healthy and anti-inflammatory, deliver bonus nutrients and antioxidants. Each of your three daily meals includes one serving of plant-based fat, from one of six categories: oils, nuts and seeds, olives, avocado, coconut, and dark chocolate.

One plant-based fat serving equals
- 1 tablespoon oil (see the following list) or oil-based pesto
- 2 tablespoons nuts or seeds (see the following list), or all-natural nut or seed butters, including tahini
- 2 tablespoons olive tapenade
- 10 green or black olives
- ¼ of a medium avocado
- 2 tablespoons unsweetened shredded or flaked coconut
- 1 ounce dark chocolate (at least 70 percent cacao)

Nuts, seeds, and butters made from them include

Almonds	Hempseeds	Pumpkin seeds
Brazil nuts	Macadamia nuts	Sesame seeds
Cashews	Peanuts	Sunflower seeds
Chia seeds	Pecans	Walnuts
Filberts (hazelnuts)	Pine nuts	
Flaxseed	Pistachios	

Oils nclude

Almond	High-oleic	Pesto (preferably
Avocado	safflower seed	vegan, made from
Cashew	High-oleic	any of the oils listed)
Coconut	sunflower seed	Pine nut
Flaxseed	Macadamia	Pistachio
Grapeseed	Olive	Pumpkin seed
Hazelnut	Peanut	Sesame seed/tahini
Hempseed	Pecan	Walnut

••

HOW TO GET A DAILY CHOCOLATE FIX

If you're a fan of my previous two weight-loss books, you're probably wondering where dark chocolate fits into this plan. Don't worry, it's right here, listed as a plant-based fat. While I opted not to make it mandatory in this plan, you can certainly include it as a plant-based fat up to once a day if you'd like. In chapter 5, you'll find recipes that include chocolate, such as Cherry Chocolate Green Goddess Smoothie (page 160), and Banana Chia Chocolate Parfait (page 137), but you can also incorporate dark chocolate in other ways. For example, if you're creating your own meals, using the DIY wardrobe design, you can leave the fat out of one meal and enjoy an ounce of dark chocolate as a postmeal treat.

••

Accessory Options

This section lists the energy accessory options. In each of your three daily meals, you'll include one serving of an energy accessory or half servings of two of these foods. However, if your energy needs are higher, you may need to add extra accessories to some or all of your meals. To find out, take the My Energy Needs quiz on page 87.

Energy Accessory Option: Whole Grain

Whole grains are a key source of vitamins, minerals, fiber, and disease-fighting antioxidants, and research shows that their consumption is tied to a lower risk of heart disease, stroke, cancer, diabetes, and obesity.

To be considered whole, a grain must contain the entire kernel, which has three distinct parts: the bran (the outer skin of the kernel), the germ (the inner part of the kernel that will sprout into a new plant), and the endosperm (the germ's food supply and largest portion of the kernel). Leaving the entire grain intact preserves the grain's vitamins, minerals, antioxidants, and fiber. This means that not only are whole grains more nutritious than refined grains, which have been stripped of their bran and germ portions, they're also more filling. When you choose a whole grain as your energy accessory, include one serving.

FACT   Of all the grains Americans eat, only about 11 percent of them are whole grains.

One whole-grain serving equals
- ½ cup cooked whole grain, such as brown rice or quinoa
- ¼ cup dry (uncooked) flaked whole grain, like rolled oats or rye flakes
- 1 cup puffed whole grain, such as puffed brown rice or millet

- 1 serving (according to the package) unsweetened hot or cold cereal, such as unsweetened organic corn flakes or five-grain hot cereal
- 3 cups popped popcorn

Whole grains include

Amaranth*

Barley

Buckwheat*

Bulgur

Corn*

Farro

Kamut

Millet*

Oats**

Quinoa*

Rice (black, brown, red, wild)*

Rye

Sorghum*

Spelt

Teff*

Triticale

Wheat berries

*Indicates gluten-free whole grains
**Indicates gluten free if not contaminated with gluten in processing—
  look for brands labeled "gluten free"

Limit These Convenience Whole-Grain Options

One hundred percent whole-grain versions of the foods listed on the following page can count as your whole-grain energy accessory, but these foods are more processed than their counterparts listed above. As a result, they tend to contain more additives and higher amounts of sodium, and they may pack more carbohydrate per serving than a cooked single whole grain, like brown rice or quinoa.

For these reasons, I recommend relying on them less often.

- 1 standard loaf-size slice of 100 percent whole-grain bread
- ½ of a 100 percent whole-grain English muffin or pita
- 2 taco-size organic whole-corn tortillas
- ½ cup cooked 100 percent whole-grain pasta or couscous
- 1 serving (according to the package) of 100 percent whole-grain crackers

SHOULD I GO GLUTEN FREE?

I opted not to make this plan entirely gluten free because I don't believe that everyone needs to avoid gluten, a protein found in some grains, including barley, rye, and wheat. To learn more about who should omit grains containing gluten and how to tell if you might have a gluten sensitivity, see page 275.

WHY YOU SHOULD CHOOSE ORGANIC CORN

I'm a huge fan of corn. It's a member of the whole-grain family, and research shows it packs more antioxidants than fruits and veggies! But more than 85 percent of U.S. corn contains genetically modified organisms (GMOs). To avoid exposure to GMOs (learn more about why this in important on page 105), look for USDA-certified organic corn products, which by law must be GMO free, or look for corn products that state that they're non-GMO.

 Foods labeled "multigrain," "100 percent wheat," "cracked wheat," or "bran" may not be whole grain products. To avoid getting tricked, look for products marked "100 percent whole grain."

Energy Accessory Option: Starchy Vegetable

Starchy vegetables are veggies that naturally contain less water and a higher amount of carbohydrate per serving than other vegetables. Many weight-loss plans omit these foods, but I think that's a shame, because like other veggies, they're rich sources of nutrients and antioxidants. They're also some of my favorite foods (hello, potatoes and squash!). To avoid carb overload, just be sure to limit yourself to one serving of these veggies as an energy accessory (or combine a half serving with a half serving of another energy accessory option).

One starchy vegetable serving equals

- ½ cup cooked starchy vegetable, such as cooked potatoes or winter squash
- 1 cup starchy vegetable that is commonly consumed raw, such as carrots or jicama
- 1 cup cooked spaghetti squash

Starchy vegetables include

Beets	Pumpkin
Carrots	Rutabagas
Celeriac	Sweet potatoes
Jicama	Turnips
Leeks	Winter squash (all varieties)
Parsnips	Yams
Potatoes (all varieties, skin-on)	

MY NEW FAVORITE ENERGY ACCESSORY

Potatoes are my number one can't-live-without starchy food, and while I typically go for fingerling or red potatoes, I have a new obsession that's becoming quite trendy: purple sweet potatoes. I first tried them at a produce show, and in addition to being gorgeous, with a flesh color that resembles the petals of an iris, they are incredibly rich and creamy. They're also versatile, as they're delicious hot or chilled. Look for them in your local supermarket, and for an easy way to prepare them, see page 174.

Energy Accessory Option: Fruit

Fruits are chock full of essential vitamins and minerals, in addition to fiber and antioxidants. But cup for cup, they do pack roughly four times more carbohydrate than veggies, about the same amount per serving as whole grains, starchy vegetables, and pulses. For this reason, I chose to include them as energy accessories.

In my private practice, I noticed that clients who included both a serving of whole grain and one of fruit sometimes would wind up with more carbohydrate than their bodies needed based on their activity levels. These clients wanted to lose weight, but they also wanted to eat something like oatmeal with fruit for breakfast, even if they were going to be sitting at a desk all morning. The solution was to include half portions of each—the halfsies strategy in this plan. This strategy is also a win-win if you enjoy having a little fruit as a sweet treat at the end of your meal, but you don't want to consume a surplus of starch.

One fruit serving equals
- 1 cup fresh or frozen fruit
- 1 medium piece fruit, about the size of a baseball
- ½ cup canned fruit packed in natural juice (no added sugar) or unsweetened pureed fruit (such as unsweetened applesauce)
- ¼ cup dried fruit, preservative free, unsweetened or sweetened with 100 percent fruit juice

Fruits include

Apples	Cantaloupe	Cranberries
Apricots	Cape gooseberries	Dates
Bananas	Casaba melon	Elderberries
Blackcurrants	Cherimoya	Figs
Blackberries	Cherries	Grapefruit
Boysenberries	Clementines	Grapes

Guavas

Honeydew melon

Jackfruit

Jujubes

Kiwano melon

Kiwis

Kumquats

Loganberries

Loquats

Lychees

Mangos

Mulberries

Nectarines

Oranges

Papayas

Passion fruit

Peaches

Pears

Persimmons

Pineapple

Plums

Pomegranates

Pummelo

Quince

Raspberries

Red currants

Star fruit

Strawberries

Tangelos

Tangerines

Watermelon

Yuzu

FACT While lemons, limes, and key limes are members of the fruit family, we don't typically bite into them, like we do apples, or enjoy them like sweeter forms of citrus, such as tangerines. For this reason, I tend to think of them as seasonings rather than fruit options. Add slices to your flat or sparkling water and tea, and squeeze a wedge or two into guacamole, hummus, garden salads, and seafood.

PICK YOUR OWN FRUIT!

One of my favorite memories as a kid is visiting an apple orchard in upstate New York to gather my very own bushel of fruit, an activity I still greatly look forward to today when visiting my family. Picking your own fruit is a great way to enjoy nature, fit in some physical activity, connect with your food, and have fun! To find out where the pick-your-own farms are in your area, check out www.pickyourown.org or www.localharvest.org.

Energy Accessory Option: Pulse

Remember, pulses serve double duty: while you can choose one serving of pulse as the energy accessory in a meal, pulses also count as a lean protein option. So I have already listed them in that section, on page 68. When they serve as energy accessories, the same types and amounts apply.

Seasonings: The Jewelry in Your Diet Wardrobe

Seasonings are another example of how well a wardrobe analogy fits. Just as you can't make an outfit out of jewelry alone, seasonings don't make a meal. Plus, though jewelry adds pizzazz to an outfit, too much takes away from a look, and sometimes it's not needed at all. For these reasons, seasonings are not a mandatory part of each meal, but I strongly encourage you to use them. Herbs and spices add flavor and aroma to meals. They're potent sources of antioxidants, and research shows that they can help rev up your metabolism and boost satiety. I've incorporated natural seasonings into most of the meals in chapter 5, and I include my favorites in the following list. However, when building your own meals, especially on the go, it's okay to omit them.

Allspice

Anise

Apple pie spice

Basil

Bay leaf

Black cardamom

Cajun seasoning

Caraway

Cardamom

Celery seed

Chiles/hot peppers (fresh
   and dried, all varieties)

Chili powder

Chive

Cilantro

Cinnamon

Citrus (juice and zest)

Clove

Coriander

Crushed red pepper flakes

Cumin

Curry spice

Dill

Garlic

Ginger

Harissa

Herbes de Provence

Horseradish

Italian herbs

Kaffir lime

Lavender

Lemongrass

Lemon verbena

Marjoram

Mint (peppermint or
  spearmint)

Mustard (wet and ground)

Nutmeg

Oregano

Paprika

Parsley

Peppercorn

Poppy seed

Pumpkin pie spice

Rosemary

Saffron

Sage

Savory

Tarragon

Tea, loose leaf (all varieties)

Thyme

Turmeric

Vanilla

Vinegar (all varieties)

Wasabi

Note: All seasoning mixes, such as Italian herbs and herbes de Provence, should be salt free.

GINGER

This aromatic spice possesses strong anti-inflammatory properties, and as I shared on page 23, inflammation is a condition related to obesity as well as numerous diseases and aging. A study of more than 250 people with osteoarthritis of the knee demonstrates its potent effects. Those who received ginger extract twice a day experienced less pain and needed fewer pain-killing meds than those who received a placebo. This may be because ginger shares some of the same pharmacological properties as nonsteroidal anti-inflammatory drugs (NSAIDs), like ibuprofen and naproxen. Ginger has also been shown to reduce muscle pain and alleviate asthma symptoms, and it's long been used to soothe the digestive tract, as a remedy for motion sickness, morning sickness, and general nausea. In addition, animal and laboratory research has shown that natural substances in ginger halt the growth of colon-cancer cells and cause ovarian cancer cells to die.

What to look for:

I highly recommend using fresh grated ginger. Not only does fresh ginger taste and smell so much better than dried ginger, but it also contains higher levels of anti-inflammatory compounds. You'll find fresh gingerroot in the produce section of your supermarket. Before you grate it, simply scrape off the delicate skin with a vegetable peeler or the edge of a spoon. Then grate it using a Microplane (one of my favorite kitchen tools) or a fine grater. Store leftover gingerroot in the refrigerator in a sealable container.

DAILY PULSE CHEAT SHEET	
Your Diet Wardrobe	
Basic meal structure—three meals per day	Each meal includes • Lean protein: 1 serving • Veggies: 1 or 2 servings • Plant-based fat: 1 serving • Energy accessory: 1 serving or 2 half servings (choose from: whole grain or starchy vegetable or fruit or pulse)
Daily pulse rule—at least one daily meal must include a pulse serving	Use the above meal structure and amounts and choose from pulse as the lean protein *or* pulse as the energy accessory

Serving sizes	Lean protein— 1 serving equals	½ cup cooked pulses (beans, peas, lentils)
		¼ cup unsweetened pea protein powder
		6 ounces nonfat organic Greek yogurt
		½ cup organic egg whites or 1 whole organic egg and 3 whites
		½ cup organic nonfat cottage cheese
		¼ cup organic nonfat ricotta cheese
		3 ounces poultry or seafood
	Veggies— 1 serving equals	1 cup fresh or frozen
		¼ cup dried, such as sundried tomatoes
		½ cup 100 percent vegetable juice
	Plant-based fat— 1 serving equals	1 tablespoon oil or oil-based pesto
		2 tablespoons nuts, seeds, or all natural nut or seed butters
		2 tablespoons olive tapenade
		10 green or black olives
		¼ medium avocado
		2 tablespoons unsweetened shredded coconut
		1 ounce dark chocolate (at least 70 percent cacao)
	Whole grain— 1 serving equals	½ cup cooked whole grain, such as brown rice or quinoa
		¼ cup dry (uncooked) flaked whole grain, like rolled oats or rye flakes
		1 cup puffed whole grain, such as puffed brown rice or millet
		1 serving (according to the package) unsweetened hot or cold cereal, such as unsweetened organic corn flakes or five-grain hot cereal
		3 cups popped popcorn
		1 standard loaf-size slice of 100 percent whole-grain bread
		½ 100 percent whole-grain English muffin or pita
		2 taco-size organic whole-corn tortillas
		½ cup cooked 100 percent whole-grain pasta or couscous
		1 serving (according to the package) 100 percent whole-grain crackers
	Starchy vegetable— 1 serving equals	½ cup cooked starchy vegetable, such as cooked potatoes or squash
		1 cup starchy vegetable that is commonly consumed raw, such as carrots or jicama
		1 cup cooked spaghetti squash
	Fruit— 1 serving equals	1 cup fresh or frozen fruit
		1 medium piece fruit, about the size of a baseball
		½ cup canned fruit packed in natural juice (no added sugar) or unsweetened pureed fruit
		¼ cup dried fruit, preservative free, unsweetened or sweetened with 100 percent fruit juice
	Pulse— 1 serving equals	½ cup cooked beans or lentils
		¼ cup unsweetened pea protein powder

Picture Your Portions

At home, I still like to measure my servings, just to double-check myself, particularly for foods that are challenging to eyeball, like oil and nut butter, and those that are carb-dense, like cooked rice and potatoes. But I don't want you to have to carry around a set of measuring cups and spoons (I certainly don't), and it's just not practical to measure everything you eat three times a day. That's why it's helpful to have a visual concept for various serving sizes. The common household objects below are items you've likely seen many times and may have around your house right now. Become familiar with them, so when you're dining out, you can visually adjust your portions to fall in line with the plan. For example, if a restaurant serves you a chicken breast that looks like the size of two smartphones, cut it in half and take half home. Or if you're spooning cut fruit onto your plate from a buffet, aim for the amount that would represent a baseball or tennis ball.

1 cup = a baseball or tennis ball

¼ cup = a golf ball

3 ounces = a deck of cards, smartphone, or checkbook

1 tablespoon = your thumb, from where it bends to the tip

Do I Need More Than One Energy Accessory?

When I developed this plan, I used my experience with private practice clients, in addition to nutrition science calculators, to determine the suitable number of servings per day from various food groups, based on the needs of an average middle-aged American woman. But your needs may differ, particularly if you're a man, taller or younger than average, or highly active. While the quiz and rules that follow are no substitute for a custom-tailored plan, they can help you adjust your meal portions to better serve your body's needs. To find out if you need additional energy accessories in your meals, answer the ten questions in this quiz.

QUIZ: MY ENERGY NEEDS

Give yourself 1 point for every *yes* response:

☐ Are you a man, or are you a woman who is over 5 feet 4 inches?

☐ Do you have more than 50 pounds to lose?

☐ Does your job require standing or moving for four or more hours per day?

☐ Do you fit in cardio-type exercise more than thirty minutes per day at least five days per week?

☐ Do you strength-train at least twice per week?

☐ Would you describe your physique as muscular?

☐ Are you under forty years of age?

☐ Would you describe your metabolism as fast (you lose weight easily)?

☐ Do you work irregular hours (not on a set schedule) or shifts other than 9 to 5?

☐ Would you describe yourself as fidgety (you never sit still, you're always animated or tapping your toe or talking with your hands)?

Score: _____

If you scored

0 to 4 points—A low score indicates that the current plan is likely adequate for your needs. However, please see the Two Additional Accessory Rules below.

5 to 6 points—This score indicates that you may need to double-accessorize some of your meals. For example, instead of selecting one serving of whole grain or starchy vegetables or fruit or pulse as the accessory

CONTINUED ON PAGE 90

My Story

Dionne Liddiard, age 43

Lost 16 pounds and 14.5 inches

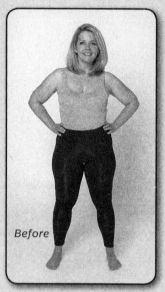

Before

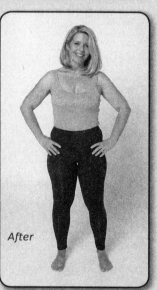

After

I've been on other diets in the past, including low-carb programs and cleanses, and like many women, I've constantly been up and down on the scale. This plan taught me that I *can* lose weight while eating whole grains, starches, and fruit, and it's an approach I can stick with! I now feel like I know how to put together a balanced meal, and I've added more vegetables to my day, especially at breakfast. I also cook healthier now for my whole family, which is so important as a married mom of four.

I'm definitely happier when I am in control of my eating, and throughout the thirty days I felt like I was completely in control. My skin looks better and the dark circles under my eyes are gone. I never had any gas despite everyone saying that beans give you gas!

When I first started I was ready to lose weight, so I wanted something that would jump start me. I like the simplicity of eating the same exact thing every day for four days and knowing that it was balanced. The pudding was a little strong on day one, but then I began to enjoy it more each day. I also liked being able to make the pudding into a smoothie. I preferred it as a smoothie in the morning, because I drink smoothies for breakfast quite often, and I liked the added volume from the water and ice. It was also great to be able to make the pudding ahead of time, and I was able to take it on the go, which helped me stay on track. I'm not sure I could have done it much longer than four days, LOL, but I was so happy with my results—seven pounds in four days!

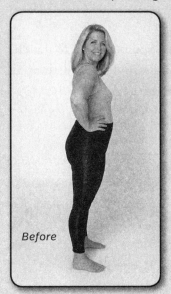

Before

In the Daily Pulse phase I really liked the Roasted Vegetable "Lasagna" and the Turkey and Veggie "Chili." I also liked being able to make extra meals in advance, and the ease of just being able to combine beans and sautéed veggies with quinoa, with a drizzle of balsamic vinegar, or dollop of pico de gallo for flavor. This plan is laid out in a way that allowed me to easily remember what a meal should contain. I also really like being able to choose my own energy accessory because it gives me the choice to go with what I'm craving. I think it was so smart to leave the energy accessory out of the recipes, but I like that there are suggestions. The desserts also make this plan so doable.

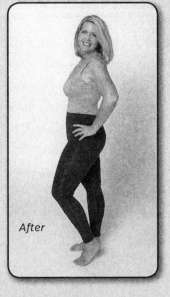

After

My favorite thing about this approach is that I feel like it is balanced, and I'm not on some crazy diet where I give up a whole food category. I feel great, and I'm happy with the amount of weight I was able to lose in thirty days. I can definitely see myself using this strategy as a way of life!

(or half servings of two of these), choose two full accessory servings, such as ½ cup of brown rice *and* 1 cup of fresh fruit. You may only need to double-accessorize in the meals prior to your most active hours. In other words, if you stand and move a lot at work, but you watch TV or sit in front of the computer at night, you may need to double-accessorize only meals 1 and 2. However, see the Two Additional Accessory Rules below for more information.

7 to 10 points—A high score indicates that you may need to double-accessorize all three of your daily meals and possibly add a fourth meal. For more information, see the Two Additional Accessory Rules below.

Two Additional Accessory Rules

In addition to what the previous quiz indicates, there are two more rules you should follow to adjust this plan to your needs.

Listen to Your Body

Each of your meals should leave you feeling satisfied, energized, nourished, and full but not overly full or stuffed. In addition, physical signs and symptoms of hunger should not return sooner than four hours after each meal. If you experience physical hunger signals, like a growling stomach, more than an hour before your scheduled meal, use a trial-and-error approach to tweak your plan. For example, perhaps one and a half energy accessories, rather than one, is just enough to keep you full and energized until your next scheduled meal. Or if you're a tall man with an active job, you may need a fourth meal each day, with the exact same structure as the other three. If that's the case, your four meals may be spaced about four hours apart, such as 7 A.M., 11 A.M., 3 P.M., and 7 P.M.

Add Accessories to Fuel Exercise

Starchy foods, aka energy accessories, fuel activity, so if you're planning to exercise or you know you're going to be more active than usual, add extra accessories to the meal prior to that activity. For example, if you work out in the morning but sit at a desk the rest of the day, double-accessorize meal 1. Or if you're planning a long afternoon walk, hike, or bike ride with your family on the weekend, double-accessorize meal 2. If you're going to be doing something physical all day, like moving into a new home, double-accessorize all three meals. It's perfectly okay to make these kinds of adjustments from meal to meal and day to day. In fact, it just makes sense based on how your body works.

Also, since most of us tend to be inactive for long stretches of the day, it's much more practical to start with a meal design based on less activity (for example, the three diet wardrobe staples plus one energy accessory per meal) and add to it than to start with a plan that contains more than your body needs and have to scale back. To use another wardrobe analogy, it makes sense to add a scarf and hat to your outfit if you're going to be outdoors in chilly weather, but it doesn't make sense to keep them on once you're inside a toasty, heated room.

• •

WHY YOU SHOULDN'T SKIP THE ENERGY ACCESSORY

You may be tempted to ditch the energy accessories—low-carb diets are still very popular—but don't. In addition to lacking energy, you're likely to have a general sense of not feeling "done" after eating. You may have lingering thoughts about food, which may prompt you to overeat (in other words, major overaccessorizing!) or to give up on losing weight altogether. But that's not the only reason to include a healthy, carb-rich food in each meal. Skipping the starch can cause your body to burn the lean protein in your meal for fuel, in place of the energy accessory you did not eat. That means the protein won't be used to maintain, build, and heal your body's protein tissues, which can negatively impact your metabolism.

WHY A MEAL-BUILDING STRATEGY IS A MUST

When you're trying to lose weight and eat healthfully, you *have* to have a strategy for how to put your meals together. Otherwise, social, environmental, and emotional triggers will take over and determine if, what, and how much you eat. With a concrete meal structure— the three-piece diet wardrobe plus an energy accessory—you can immediately see how far off course you'd end up if you gave in to eating, say, a stuffed burrito or a mound of pasta. But keep in mind that having a concrete meal structure isn't about restriction. A meal-building plan simply provides a guiding principle to ensure that you don't fall short of or exceed your body's needs. Like wardrobe rules, it just makes sense!

[4]

The Power of Pulses

Each year the average American consumes 74 pounds of red meat—the amount of beef in 296 quarter-pound burgers. We eat 23 pounds of cheese, more than quadruple what Americans ate in the 1950s. And nearly half of all Americans drink soda *every single day*.

Yet on any given day, only 14 percent of Americans eat pulses. On a yearly basis, we average just 6½ pounds of pulses—that's pinto beans, black beans, kidney beans, navy beans, chickpeas, and lentils *combined*. That's nothing!

Today Americans eat about one-third fewer pulses than we did half a century ago and dramatically less than folks eat today in Latin America, India, and Africa. Pulses are staples in those regions. Red lentil stew, spiced lentil dip, lentil soup, red bean and sweet potato stew, green lentil curry, savory hummus—you can't count the number of delicious pulse-based recipes adored worldwide.

Health authorities in Brazil are so sold on pulses that the country's food pyramid singles out beans as a food group that should be consumed daily. I couldn't agree more. Incorporating pulses into your daily diet is the cornerstone of my plan. In this chapter, I share some of the incredible research that explains why pulses are the best-kept secret to protecting your health and shedding pounds and inches—and keeping them off.

The Study That Sparked My Plan

Many "diets" these days are based on cutting out entire food groups, like all carbs, including whole grains, fruit, and many vegetables. My clients find these diets restrictive and frustrating; they just reinforce the idea that weight loss is about deprivation. But it doesn't have to be. Plenty of research shows you can lose weight by *adding* foods to your diet rather than taking foods away. This is the kind of research my clients love to hear about, because it makes losing weight seem within reach.

It was one of these "add a food" studies, published in the *British Journal of Nutrition,* that sparked my entire pulse plan. Scientists at the University of Toronto divided overweight and obese volunteers into two groups. One group was asked to do nothing more than add 5 cups of pulses—including lentils, chickpeas, navy beans, and yellow peas—to their diets each week for eight weeks. The other group was simply counseled to eat 500 fewer calories a day. After two months, both groups had lost weight, even though the pulse eaters weren't asked to cut calories. What's more, levels of HDL cholesterol, the type that protects against heart disease, increased among the pulse group and dropped among the calorie cutters. Blood sugar levels decreased in both groups, but the drop among the pulse eaters was nearly four times greater!

To me, this study scored a triple "Wow!" First, the pulse group lost as much weight as the other group by *adding* a food—without even attempting to cut calories. Second, the pulse eaters added a food rich in carbs, something typically vilified by dieters. Third, adding pulses triggered better cholesterol readings and significantly lower blood sugar levels (which, as I explain on page 24, is critical for weight control). My interest piqued, I began collecting studies about pulses, and the wows kept coming. I discovered far more research than I could fit into this chapter, but to give you a taste of why I'm so besotted with beans, lentils, and peas, I have summarized my ten favorite studies about pulses and weight loss and sprinkled in other research about the power of pulses.

Eat Pulses, Lose Weight: Ten Impressive Studies

In short, studies convincingly show that this deliciously satisfying group of foods can accomplish the following:

- Trigger weight loss
- Regulate appetite
- Lower diabetes risk
- Increase heart health
- Protect against cancer
- Improve athletic performance
- Enhance overall nutrition

Pulses Quadruple Weight Loss

Scientists at Indiana's Purdue University and Bastyr University in Washington State asked volunteers to consume 30 percent fewer calories than usual, randomly assigning the dieters to one of three eating plans. The first plan included 3 cups of beans and lentils per week, the second included nearly 2 cups of pulses a day for women and 3 for men, and the third involved eating minimal amounts of pulses. After six weeks, all three groups lost weight, but the dieters who consumed the most pulses shed the most pounds. The thrice-weekly bean/lentil eaters lost 7.5 pounds, those on the pulse-loaded diet lost 8.5 pounds, and those with the minimal pulse intake lost just 2 pounds.

Pulses Offer Heart Protection Plus Weight Loss

In a study published in the *European Journal of Nutrition,* thirty obese adults were randomly assigned to one of two calorie-restricted diets for eight weeks. One diet contained no beans or lentils; the other contained four weekly servings of lentils, chickpeas, peas, or beans. The pulse eaters lost more weight—17 pounds compared to 11—and experienced greater improvements in cholesterol and blood pressure. They also had a greater reduction in C-reactive protein (CRP). As I noted on page 23, CRP is a blood marker for inflammation, a known trigger of premature aging, heart disease, type 2 diabetes, and obesity.

Pulses Attack Belly Fat

One of my favorite studies, from the *British Journal of Nutrition,* tracked overweight women with high cholesterol who, twice a day for twenty-eight days, received muffins containing either whole pea flour (equivalent to ½ cup of pulses), fractionated pea flour (pea hulls only), or white wheat flour. At the end of the study, the women who ate the muffins with whole pea protein powder had the lowest waist-to-hip ratios, indicating that fat was directed away from the waistline. Previous animal research compared rats fed an unhealthy diet with or without added chickpeas to rodents that chowed down on healthy fare. The chickpea-eating rats had significantly reduced belly fat and had blood sugar and insulin levels similar to the animals fed healthy food.

· ·

ANOTHER REASON PULSES REDUCE BELLY FAT

A study from Wake Forest Baptist Medical Center found that for every 10-gram increase in soluble fiber eaten daily, belly fat was reduced by 3.7 percent over five years. Soluble fiber is the type of fiber that absorbs water to form a gel-like texture (for example, the stickiness of oatmeal after you add water). Pulses are a top source of soluble fiber. Of the 6 grams of fiber in ½ cup of cooked black beans, about 2.5 are of the soluble variety.

· ·

Pulses Boost Feelings of Fullness and Reduce Snack Attacks

In a French study, researchers offered participants a version of shepherd's pie made with either potato or bean puree. After the potato meal, the participants' blood glucose levels rose sharply, peaking thirty to forty-five minutes after eating and then falling *below* their initial blood sugar levels two to three hours later. In contrast, the bean eaters experienced a slow, steady increase in blood sugar. Three hours later they reported less hunger. Four hours after the meal they reported a significantly lower desire to snack.

Pulse Eaters Eat More but Weigh Less

Data from the National Nutrition and Health Examination Survey found that adults who regularly eat beans consume about 200 more calories daily than those who don't, yet they weigh on average 6.6 pounds less. These results were even more dramatic for teenagers: those who ate beans consumed 335 more daily calories but weighed 7.3 pounds less than teens who shunned beans. The report also found that adult bean eaters had smaller waistline measurements than bean avoiders.

Pea Protein Beats Whey at Suppressing Hunger

Dutch researchers gave overweight men and women beverages made with either pea protein or whey protein to test the effect of these drinks on appetite. The pea protein version delayed the return of hunger by up to twenty-three minutes longer than the whey drink. In addition, after four hours the pulse drinkers felt less hungry than those who drank the whey beverage.

Pulses Rival a High-Protein Diet for Weight Loss— With Bonus Heart Protection

Spanish researchers tested the effects of various protein sources on changes in mitochondria, the fuel producing engines inside your cells that burn calories. Thirty-five obese men were randomly assigned to a high-protein diet or a diet with either added pulses or fatty fish. The high-protein and pulse diets resulted in the greatest weight loss, with nearly identical results. These two diets also triggered the greatest change in mitochondria, indicating a boost in metabolic rate. But only the pulse group experienced a drop in LDL cholesterol, the type linked to heart disease, our nation's number one killer of both men and women.

Pulses Boost Satiety and Curb Cravings for Processed Snacks

Australian researchers asked forty-two volunteers to consume their usual diets plus about 3½ ounces of chickpeas daily for twelve weeks and then return to their typical diets for another month. Based on food diaries, the participants ate less from every food group, especially grains, during the three-month chickpea intervention. They also reported feeling more satisfied during the chickpea experiment. In the four weeks after the study ended, their intake of processed snacks spiked.

A High-Fiber Bean Diet Rivals a Low-Carb Diet for Weight Loss

Researchers at Loma Linda University randomly assigned 173 overweight women and men to either a fiber-rich, bean-enhanced diet or a low-carbohydrate diet. Low-carb dieters lost just 2 more pounds over sixteen weeks, but only the bean eaters experienced reductions in LDL choles-

ANOTHER REASON TO REACH FOR PULSES—MEAT AND CHEESE FOUND TO BE AS HARMFUL AS SMOKING!

A recent study from the University of Southern California, which tracked a large sample of adults for nearly two decades, found that eating a diet rich in animal-based protein during middle age was tied to a fourfold increase in the likelihood of dying of cancer compared to those who consumed a diet low in animal protein—a mortality risk comparable to that of smoking! The researchers also found that middle-aged men and women under the age of sixty-five who eat high amounts of animal protein—including meat, milk, and cheese—were more susceptible to early death from any cause. In fact, animal protein lovers were 74 percent more likely to die earlier than those who consumed lower amounts of these foods, including death from diabetes. The study also concluded that the consumption of plant-based proteins, such as beans, did not lead to the same mortality effects as animal proteins. Once again, evidence to support the power of pulses!

terol, which as I just noted is the type that increases heart disease risk. The heart-protective effects were maintained one year later.

Pulses Boost Calorie and Fat Burning

In a study published in *Applied Physiology, Nutrition, and Metabolism,* University of Manitoba scientists found that hamsters fed diets containing 10 percent pea flour in place of cornstarch took in more oxygen, a measure of metabolic rate. Scientists believe this is because the pea-based diets contained nearly 25 percent more arginine, an amino acid that's been shown to increase both carbohydrate and fat burning. Fava beans and lentils also are rich in arginine as well as glutamine, another amino acid that in human research has been tied to a 50 percent boost in post-meal calorie burning.

All these studies convinced me that if you're trying to lose weight, particularly without fighting constant hunger, pulses *must* have a daily place in your diet. While my overall "diet wardrobe" design, laid out starting on page 84, is essential to my plan, the Daily Pulse rule is truly the cornerstone. Based on the research, I feel confident in saying that eating at least one pulse serving per day, for a minimum total of 3½ cups per week, is a savvy, cutting edge weight-loss strategy—one that will also leave you feeling satisfied and help to optimize your health.

 FACT Beans are the latest approach to helping our canine companions trim down. In a study at Colorado State University Veterinary Teaching Hospital, dogs fed powdered black and pinto beans lost more weight than those who munched the same number of pulse-free calories. The bean-eating dogs also experienced greater improvements in blood cholesterol.

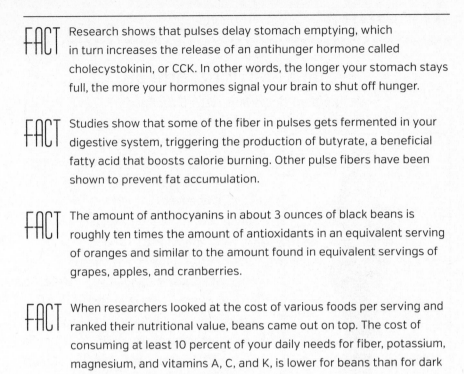

FACT   Research shows that pulses delay stomach emptying, which in turn increases the release of an antihunger hormone called cholecystokinin, or CCK. In other words, the longer your stomach stays full, the more your hormones signal your brain to shut off hunger.

FACT   Studies show that some of the fiber in pulses gets fermented in your digestive system, triggering the production of butyrate, a beneficial fatty acid that boosts calorie burning. Other pulse fibers have been shown to prevent fat accumulation.

FACT   The amount of anthocyanins in about 3 ounces of black beans is roughly ten times the amount of antioxidants in an equivalent serving of oranges and similar to the amount found in equivalent servings of grapes, apples, and cranberries.

FACT   When researchers looked at the cost of various foods per serving and ranked their nutritional value, beans came out on top. The cost of consuming at least 10 percent of your daily needs for fiber, potassium, magnesium, and vitamins A, C, and K, is lower for beans than for dark green and deep yellow veggies.

Eight Benefits of Pulses Beyond Weight Loss

Pulses do a lot more than control appetite, regulate blood sugar, and boost weight loss. Here are eight additional reasons a daily dose of pulses is vital to your overall health.

Heart Protection

Research reported in the *Archives of Internal Medicine* found that men and women who ate pulses four times per week had a 22 percent lower risk of heart disease than those who consumed pulses just once a week.

CONTINUED ON PAGE 104

My Story

Yadira Martinez, age 39

Lost 14 pounds and 18.5 inches

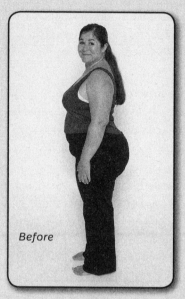

Before

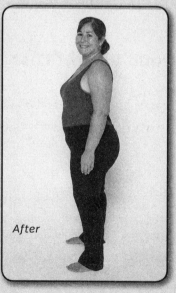

After

I have been seriously overweight for the last fifteen to sixteen years. I was always looking for the magic pill to lose weight. Whenever I tried to lose weight I would lose a pound only to gain back three, and when I wasn't trying to lose I had no restrictions or self-control. I thought if I had a serving of vegetables then it was okay to have a gazillion candies. I always found ways to justify my overindulgences. My saying was "if it's sweet, salty, and/or fried, then it's for me."

This opportunity came about at the right time for me. What I really needed was realistic limits, and that's just what this plan gave me. The Rapid Pulse was challenging, but I was so happy that I hung in there. I lost 8 pounds, and my first meal on day five, the Mexi Omelet, was astonishingly satisfying and delicious. I felt like I was eating a lot of food!!! If I had started the Daily Pulse immediately, I probably would have found the plan unsatisfying and bland, and the portion size might have been not enough. I think the Rapid Pulse really did reset my system. Flavors became more prominent (I can actually taste the sweetness in tomatoes!), and I'm now eating less because I can pay attention and stop when I'm full. I feel as if the Rapid Pulse cleansed and refreshed my palate!

The Daily Pulse taught me that food doesn't need to drenched in salt or fried to taste good. The Chilled Turkey Pesto Salad and the Pineapple Ginger Coconut Parfait were my favorite meals (I was happier than a pig in mud when I ate the parfaits). And the Turkey and Veggie "Chili" was amazing.

My husband also lost weight without even completely following the plan, and my five-year-old daughter saw the importance of eating veggies, since they were in all our meals. When I made the Savory Turkey Stuffed Zucchini my daughter ate a whole zucchini without complaining!

This plan just got easier and easier to follow. I also like the fact that I'm able to modify my "own" recipes. And I ate at restaurants often and was still able to get great results. I even went to a fair and was able to choose foods like grilled chicken with peppers and onions and corn on the cob. This strategy is so easy to follow. I could go practically anywhere and stick with the "wardrobe"—I had lots of options.

Toward the end of the thirty days I felt so motivated I went for a run. I haven't done that since I was in high school! This from a woman who used to get tired sweeping and mopping the floors. Now that's a breeze!

My digestive system also benefitted greatly from this plan. And I noticed a difference in my skin—it's clearer—and I have a healthy glow to go along with it. I think I look younger! This experience also taught me that I don't have to turn to food as a way to deal with difficult situations or life. Sure, boatloads of carbs taste mighty fine, but I was able to survive without them!

I plan to continue eating this way. And if I do have a slice of pizza, it will be thin whole-wheat crust with lots of veggies and perhaps a smidge of cheese. And it will be an occasional treat—such a different perspective than I had before! This is only the beginning. I know I'll keep going!

Breast Cancer Protection

Harvard researchers analyzed data from over ninety thousand women ages twenty-six to forty-six who participated in the Nurses Health Study II. After eight years, scientists found that the women who ate beans or lentils at least twice a week were 24 percent less likely to develop breast cancer than women who consumed them less than once a month.

In a study on rats, scientists at Colorado State University examined the anticancer activity of six types of beans, including small red, great northern, navy, black, dark red, and white kidney beans. The rats that consumed every type of bean had a 30 percent lower incidence of breast cancer than the rats that ate no beans. The bean-fed rats also had fewer than half the number of malignant tumors than the rats fed the normal diet.

Reduced Diabetes Risk

In a study published in *Archives of Internal Medicine,* University of Toronto researchers randomly assigned 121 patients with type 2 diabetes to one of two diets for three months. One diet contained 1 cup of pulses per day. The other was bolstered with insoluble fiber from wheat grain. The pulse diet was not only more effective at improving blood sugar control but also significantly lowered blood pressure.

Reduced Colon Cancer Risk

Among nearly thirty-five thousand women, those who ate four or more servings of pulses each week reduced their risk of developing colon cancer by one-third. And in people previously diagnosed with colon cancer, increasing bean consumption has been shown to slash the risk of recurrence up to 45 percent.

Enhanced Athletic Endurance

You may not think of pulses as an optimal pre-exercise food, but Greek researchers found that they're effective endurance boosters. Scientists served athletes either lentils or potatoes and then put them through a treadmill workout. For five minutes the athletes ran at 60 percent of their maximum intensity levels, then they ran for forty-five minutes at 70 percent of their max. Finally, they ran until exhaustion at 80 percent of their max effort. Compared to the potato eaters, the lentil eaters lasted 23 percent longer and maintained better long-term blood sugar regulation over the entire span of the workouts.

Pulses Up the Intake of Key Nutrients

In a Canadian study, researchers found that consumers who ate the most pulses had a significantly lower risk of falling short on key nutrients, including protein, fiber, thiamin, vitamin B_6, folate, potassium, zinc, and magnesium.

Most Pulses Aren't Genetically Modified Foods

GMOs, or genetically modified organisms, are plants or animals created through biotechnology gene-splicing techniques. This process is also referred to as genetic engineering, or GE. GE merges DNA from different species, creating combinations of plant, animal, bacterial, and viral genetics that do not occur in nature or through traditional crossbreeding.

Scientists and health professionals, including me, are concerned about the potential risks of consuming GMO foods, such as possible allergic reactions or intolerances and a harmful impact on agriculture and the natural balance of our ecosystems. Environmentalists are also concerned that GMOs create the potential for superweeds and superpests, weeds and bugs that become resistant to chemicals that have been used to keep them under control.

Unlike soybeans, pulses are not considered at a high risk of being GMOs. High-risk foods include genetically engineered foods that are currently in commercial production, such as alfalfa, canola, corn, cotton, papaya, soy, sugar beets, yellow summer squash, and zucchini.

Currently, U.S. consumers have no way of knowing which foods and products contain GMOs. If you'd like to avoid GMO foods, look for USDA-certified organic foods, which must contain no GM ingredients, or look for those verified by the Non-GMO Project (www.nongmoproject .org).

Pulses Are Gluten Free and Don't Cause Allergies

Not only are pulses plant based and not usually a genetically modified food, they are also gluten free, and they aren't one of the common allergens. The most common allergens, sometimes referred to as "the big eight," are milk; eggs; peanuts; tree nuts, such as almonds, cashews, and walnuts; fish; shellfish, such as shrimp, crab, lobster; soy; and wheat. Many people who battle food allergies also struggle with gluten intolerance (see page 275 for more). When you're forced to eliminate allergens and/or gluten, you lose significant nutrients. Pulses are ideal for filling these nutritional gaps.

[5]

Recipes

I had so much fun creating, testing, and fine-tuning the recipes in this book, and I'm thrilled to be sharing them with you! I've kept the ingredients and steps simple while focusing on flavor and quality, and there's something for everyone. You'll find easy, no-cook options, such as Garlic Basil White Bean Dip; hearty, aromatic selections like Moroccan Lentil Soup; crisp salads, including Spinach Walnut Salad and Chilled Chicken Dijon Salad; as well as satisfying omelets, frosty smoothies, more creamy dips, cheesy casseroles, and ethnic-inspired stir-fries and soups. All these delectable choices will help you shed pounds while feeling fantastic and enjoying meals you'll look forward to.

Before you dive into the recipes, remember there are two ways to follow this deliciously slimming plan. You can either use the wardrobe design and lists in chapter 3 to create your own meals or you can simply choose any of the flavorful recipes in this chapter that strike your fancy. Or you can combine my recipes with meals you've created on your own.

Each day you'll enjoy three satisfying, energizing meals and possibly a snack. Be sure to check the My Energy Needs quiz on page 87 to see if you need to add that snack. All the meal options in this chapter are interchangeable. In other words, they aren't categorized into breakfast, lunch, and dinner. I've chosen this approach because many of my clients enjoy starting the day with meals that seem like traditional lunch or dinner options, like a casserole, or prefer to eat an egg dish, like quiche, for dinner. That's perfectly okay.

I've listed each meal according to its protein source: eggs, dairy, poultry, seafood, or pulses.

As you learned in chapter 3, each of your three daily meals will include three diet wardrobe staples: lean protein plus veggies plus plant-based fat (think a top, a bottom, and footwear—three must-have elements). At each meal you'll also add one of four possible energy accessories:

Whole grain
or
Starchy vegetable
or
Fruit
or
Pulse

To help you get used to this meal structure, I have laid out the recipes *exactly* this way. Each delectable choice is made from a trio of lean protein, veggies, and plant-based fat (often with seasoning "jewelry"). Underneath the recipe, you'll find suggested ways to add your energy accessory. Remember, you have the option of adding a half serving of two accessories, and the choices I list below each recipe are only suggestions— feel free to choose others you may prefer. Also, depending on the results of your My Energy Needs quiz, you may need to include full portions of two energy accessories at some or all of your meals (see page 76).

Because your energy needs may vary from meal to meal or day to day, I have opted to leave the energy accessories out of each recipe. I want you to think of them as add-ons to each meal and keep them separate from your main meal prep. This way, you can choose exactly what you're in the mood for or have time for at any given meal. For example, let's say you're having the Mexi Omelet for breakfast; if you're in a rush, you can grab a slice of whole-grain toast or a Granny Smith apple or, when you have more time, you can make oven-roasted potatoes.

DOUBLE PULSING

In the pulse meals section, you'll note that doubling the pulse portion or adding another pulse serving is an option for adding your energy accessory. One of my favorite double pulse meals is the Black Bean Avocado Cilantro Hummus with a side of Oven-Roasted Chickpeas. I love to sprinkle some of the chickpeas on top of the hummus and scoop them up with the broccoli! Other days, I enjoy the hummus with fresh fruit, raw carrots, or a half portion of each. Having these choices every time you select a meal is part of the beauty of leaving the energy accessory out of the main recipe. *You* get to choose what you want to add. You also get to determine how much to add, using the My Energy Needs quiz (see page 87). After all, if you're about to go on an afternoon hike, you shouldn't eat the same meal you'd have if you were going to sit at a desk until dinner. This customization best supports your personal preferences and optimizes your metabolism, so you can maximize your weight-loss results.

Also, leaving the energy accessory out of the recipe means you can readily adjust your portion. If you need more than one serving of energy accessory because you're going to be more active than usual (see page 91), simply add more. This is a unique aspect of my plan and one reason it's so effective. As I noted on page 64, overdoing starchy foods is where most people go wrong when trying to lose weight. So it's far easier to use a meal-building strategy that lets you *add* food to a meal rather than one that requires you to take food away or leave some tasty "accessories" on your plate. And because the accessory isn't built into the recipe, you'll also cut back on food waste.

When you're selecting meals from this chapter, just don't forget rule #2: include a pulse serving in at least one daily meal. You can do this by either

- choosing a pulse as the energy accessory (the *plus-pulse* option)
  or
- choosing a meal with pulse as the lean protein (the *pulse-as-protein* option).

It's perfectly okay to enjoy more than one pulse serving each day. For example, you might choose black beans as the energy accessory with the California Omelet for meal 1 (a plus-pulse option), whip up the White Bean and Kale Soup for meal 2 (a pulse-as-protein option), and eat no pulse in meal 3. However, don't double up one day and go pulse free the next. Eating at least one pulse serving daily is essential to this plan.

Before you start exploring the recipes, I'd like you to keep three additional things in mind:

Stick to the Meal Timing Rules

Eat your first meal within an hour of waking up, eat your second meal four to five hours later, and eat your third meal four to five hours after that. See page 59 for more details on meal timing.

Customize Any Recipe with Trade-Outs

Any of my meals can easily be tweaked based on personal preferences, needs, or food availability. For example, if a meal calls for shrimp and you're allergic to shellfish or simply dislike shrimp, trade it for salmon, another fish of your choice, or even chicken or turkey. If a recipe includes broccoli and you're not a fan, replace it with a veggie you enjoy. Or if you think a recipe would work better with extra-virgin olive oil than with coconut oil, make the switch.

This trade-out rule holds true for any part of the recipe—lean protein, veggies, and plant-based fat, even seasonings. If you're looking for trade-out ideas, either to create a new version of a recipe or give my version a twist, consult the lists in chapter 3. And remember that when it comes to the energy accessory, the choice is completely up to you. The options I include below each recipe are only suggestions based on what I think pairs well. But if I've listed fingerling potatoes as the starchy vegetable accessory and you're more in the mood for butternut squash or raw carrots, go for it! This trade-out rule should make it easy for you to follow the plan based on your personal needs and favorites, and even what's in season or what's on sale. It also allows you to craft new recipes using your own creativity by simply switching up some of the ingredients. For example, you can easily turn the Savory Turkey Stuffed Zucchini recipe into Savory Chicken Stuffed Eggplant!

Check Your Mise en Place

You'll notice the recipes' ingredients are listed in this order: lean protein; vegetable; plant-based fat; seasoning suggestion. This makes it easier for you to switch categories of ingredients out, but it also means the ingredients are not necessarily listed in the order you'll use them. If this is at all confusing, try doing what chefs do: read the recipe and prepare and measure all the ingredients before you get started—this is called a *mise en place* ("placement" or "assembly"), and it's a cook's ticket to efficient meal prep.

Use On-the-Go Options
When You're Short on Time

You'll notice that the last meal in each of the sections in this chapter is an on-the-go option. I've also made the following notes next to each recipe:

- Meals that can be made ahead are marked *Make Ahead.*
- Meals that are easily portable and don't require reheating (even if the recipe indicates the dish is served warm) say *Take It with You.*
- Meals that take less than twenty minutes to make say *Quick!*
- Meals that can be frozen and reheated are marked *Freeze & Reheat.*

Look for these designations as you scan the recipes. Other strategies for saving time include the following:

- Cook frequently used ingredients, such as chicken breast and quinoa, on the weekends, and stock your fridge for use during the week.
- Buy no-added-sodium canned beans and vacuum-sealed steamed beans and lentils rather than dry versions that need to be soaked and boiled.
- Stock up on healthy frozen goods. Great options include frozen fruit, frozen organic corn, and frozen precooked shrimp. Many stores also now carry frozen pulses and whole grains.
- Use shortcut ingredients, such as instant or heat-and-eat brown and wild rice.

Okay, ready to get cooking? Have at it!

Egg-Based Meals

California Omelet—Quick!
....

Lean protein: **½ cup organic egg whites or 1 whole organic egg and 3 whites, whisked**

Vegetable: **¼ cup minced yellow onion; ¼ cup low-sodium organic vegetable broth; 1 small vine-ripened tomato, diced; ¾ cup baby spinach leaves**

Plant-based fat: **¼ medium avocado, sliced**

Seasoning suggestion: **½ teaspoon minced garlic, ¹⁄₁₆ teaspoon black pepper, ⅛ teaspoon crushed red pepper flakes**

In a medium pan over low heat, sauté the onion in the broth until it is translucent. Add the tomato, garlic, black pepper, and crushed red pepper, and sauté 2 to 3 more minutes. Remove the veggies from the pan and set them aside. Add the whisked eggs to the pan set over low heat and top the eggs with the spinach. Allow the eggs to set and then carefully fold one side over onto the other. Remove the omelet from the pan, top it with the sautéed tomato and onion, and garnish it with sliced avocado.

Energy Accessory Ideas:

Whole grain: serve with 1 slice 100 percent whole-grain toast

or

Starchy vegetable: serve with ½ cup cubed oven-roasted, skin-on red potatoes

or

Fruit: serve with 1 cup fresh fruit

or

Pulse: serve with ½ cup cooked black beans or Oven-Roasted Chickpeas (see page 175)

Mediterranean Mushroom Olive Scramble—Quick!
....

Lean protein: **½ cup organic egg whites or 1 whole organic egg and 3 whites, whisked**

Vegetable: **¼ cup minced yellow onion, ¾ cup sliced white button mushrooms**

Plant-based fat: **10 Mediterranean olives, sliced (black, green, or mixed)**

Seasoning suggestion: **¼ teaspoon salt-free Italian seasoning**

Spray a small sauté pan with olive oil–based nonstick spray and set it over low heat. Sauté the onion and mushrooms until the onion is translucent. In a small bowl, whisk the Italian seasoning into the eggs. Add the eggs and sliced olives to the pan, and using a heat-resistant spatula, push the eggs gently and continuously into the center of the pan until the eggs are cooked through. Slide the scramble onto a plate and serve.

Energy Accessory Ideas:

Whole grain: add ½ cup cooked quinoa to the scramble with the olives, or serve it on the side

or

Starchy vegetable: serve with ½ cup oven-baked fingerling potatoes or Baked Purple Sweet Potato (see page 174)

or

Fruit: serve with 1 cup fresh fruit

or

Pulse: serve with ½ cup cooked lentils

Pesto Egg Salad—*Quick!, Make Ahead, Take It with You*
....

Lean protein: **1 whole hard-boiled organic egg and 3 hard-boiled organic egg whites, chopped**
Vegetable: **¼ cup finely chopped red bell pepper, 2 tablespoons minced red onion, 3 large outer leaves romaine lettuce**
Plant-based fat: **1 tablespoon basil pesto**

In a small bowl, toss the chopped eggs with the bell pepper, onion, and pesto to coat everything thoroughly. Spoon the mixture onto the romaine leaves, roll them up, and enjoy.

Energy Accessory Ideas:

Whole grain: spread the egg salad onto 1 serving (according to the package) 100 percent whole-grain crackers or 1 slice 100 percent whole-grain bread

or

Starchy vegetable: serve with ½ cup Oven-Roasted Sweet Potato "Fries" (see page 175)

or

Fruit: serve with 1 cup fresh fruit

or

Pulse: serve with ½ cup pulse, such as Oven-Roasted Chickpeas (see page 175)

Wilted Lemon Pepper Arugula Salad—*Quick!*
....

Lean protein: **1 whole hard-boiled organic egg and 3 hard-boiled organic egg whites, chopped**
Vegetable: **1½ cups fresh arugula; ¼ cup grape tomatoes (about 8), sliced in half**
Plant-based fat: **1 tablespoon extra-virgin olive oil**

Seasoning suggestion: **2 teaspoons balsamic vinegar, 1 teaspoon fresh-squeezed lemon juice, 1 teaspoon Dijon mustard, ½ teaspoon minced garlic, ¼ teaspoon black pepper**

Whisk together the olive oil, vinegar, lemon juice, mustard, garlic, and black pepper. Toss the arugula and tomatoes with this dressing. In a sauté pan set over medium heat, quickly sauté the dressed veggies, just until the arugula begins to wilt. Transfer the mixture to a salad bowl, top it with the chopped eggs, and serve.

Energy Accessory Ideas:

Whole grain: sprinkle ½ cup cooked wild rice over the salad

or

Starchy vegetable: add ½ cup cubed oven-roasted butternut squash or Baked Purple Sweet Potato (see page 174) to the salad

or

Fruit: serve with 1 cup fresh fruit

or

Pulse: add ½ cup cooked cannellini beans to the salad

Gingery Egg Satay—*Make Ahead, Take It with You*

Lean protein: **1 whole hard-boiled organic egg and 3 hard-boiled organic egg whites, chopped**

Vegetable: **¼ cup each shredded cabbage, minced yellow onion, minced green bell pepper, and minced red bell pepper; ¼ cup low-sodium organic vegetable broth**

Plant-based fat: **2 tablespoons natural peanut butter**

Seasoning suggestion: **½ teaspoon grated fresh ginger, ½ teaspoon minced garlic, ⅛ teaspoon crushed red pepper flakes**

In a medium pan set over medium heat, simmer the cabbage, onion, and bell pepper in the broth until vegetables are tender. Combine the peanut butter, ginger, garlic, and crushed red pepper in a medium bowl. Add the vegetables and toss them to coat; add up to 1 tablespoon of water if you prefer thinner peanut sauce. Transfer the satay to a serving bowl, top it with the chopped eggs, and serve.

Energy Accessory Ideas:

Whole grain: add ½ cup cooked 100 percent whole-grain buckwheat soba noodles to the bowl with the sautéed veggies

or

Starchy vegetable: serve over 1 cup cooked spaghetti squash

or

Fruit: serve with 1 cup fresh fruit

or

Pulse: add ½ cup black-eyed peas with the egg

What Real Women Are Saying About the Plan

Joy Bennett:

*"Love, love, loved the Basil Balsamic Tuna Salad!
Very tasty and filling!"*

*"Love the Oven-Roasted Chickpeas.
I added a pinch of cayenne to give them a little kick!"*

*"The Chilled Chicken Dijon Salad tasted even better
after being in the fridge overnight!"*

*"I must say that I really like the addition of chickpeas to a salad as
my energy accessory drizzled with a little balsamic vinegar—yummy!"*

*"I couldn't wait to try the oatmeal. I was a little bit nervous
about the pea protein powder because I had never tasted it before, but
I must say I loved it. It added a nice smooth texture to the oatmeal
and was very filling. Two thumbs way up on this recipe!!!!"*

Dionne Liddiard:

*"I learned that I can do anything for four days! I thought the pudding
days flew by, and I liked not having to think about what to eat."*

*"I feel optimistic about staying on the plan. Sometimes
I get lazy on a weight program and don't give myself variety,
which probably sets me up for failure, because I get sick of eating
the same things. This time I'm going to try lots of new recipes!"*

*"I like that I can make extra meals ahead of time
so I can just grab one fast for lunch."*

"I'm staying on track, and I don't have any desire to go 'off' this plan!"

*"I was at an event with bagels and cinnamon rolls spread out
in front of me—I didn't feel tempted at all!"*

Yadira Martinez:

*"Loved the Pineapple Ginger Coconut Parfait!
I wanted to lick my bowl!"*

*"The coconut oil in the Cheesy Cauliflower Casserole made the
dish seem buttery. I was totally full and content when finished!"*

*"Having a parfait makes me feel like I'm having dessert for dinner!
It feels good to satisfy my cravings with something healthy."*

"I had never had oven-roasted chickpeas. I enjoyed the nutty taste."

Kristi Fletcher:

*"I made the Broccoli Cashew Chicken Stir-Fry for the whole
family. Everyone loved it, and it soon became a family favorite!"*

*"OMGosh! The Cherry Chocolate Green Goddess
Smoothie was delicious and flavorful!"*

*"The Moroccan Lentil Soup was so good and not
something I would normally have tried. I am seriously
loving the recipes in this book. So yum!!"*

Sandy Pinzon:

"I loved the Cheesy Cauliflower Casserole!"

Amy Canning:

*"The Basil Balsamic Tuna Salad is an awesome recipe!
I feel refreshed after eating it!"*

*"The Black Bean "Tacos" are perfectly seasoned, and so much food!
I love the combination of the flavors, and I felt energized all day long."*

*"The Broccoli Cashew Chicken Stir-Fry is one of my favorite
dinners to make. It's super easy. Love it!"*

Mexi Omelet—*Quick!*

....

Lean protein: ½ cup organic egg whites or 1 whole organic egg and 3 whites, whisked
Vegetable: ¼ cup each minced white onion, grape tomatoes sliced in half (about 8), sliced white button mushrooms, and minced green bell pepper
Plant-based fat: ¼ medium avocado
Seasoning suggestion: 1 teaspoon chopped fresh cilantro; 1 teaspoon fresh-squeezed lime juice; 1 small jalapeño, minced; ¹⁄₁₆ teaspoon black pepper

In a bowl, combine the avocado, cilantro, lime juice, jalapeño, and black pepper, and mash the mixture lightly to make guacamole; chill. Spray a small sauté pan with olive oil–based nonstick spray and place it over low heat. Sauté the onion, tomatoes, mushrooms, and bell pepper until the onion is translucent and the bell pepper is tender. Remove the veggies from the pan and set them aside. Add the eggs to the pan and allow them to just set, then carefully fold one side over onto the other. Slide the omelet onto a plate, top it with the sautéed veggies, garnish it with the guacamole, and serve.

Energy Accessory Ideas:

Whole grain: serve with ½ cup oven-roasted corn or 2 taco-size organic whole-corn tortillas
or
Starchy vegetable: serve with ½ cup cubed oven-roasted, skin-on red potatoes
or
Fruit: serve with 1 cup fresh fruit
or
Pulse: serve with ½ cup cooked black beans

Ginger Broccoli Scramble—*Quick!*

....

Lean protein: ½ cup organic egg whites or 1 whole organic egg and 3 whites, whisked
Vegetable: ¼ cup minced yellow onion, ¼ cup low-sodium organic vegetable broth, 1 cup small broccoli florets
Plant-based fat: 1 tablespoon extra-virgin coconut oil
Seasoning suggestion: ½ teaspoon minced garlic, ½ teaspoon grated fresh ginger, ⅛ teaspoon crushed red pepper flakes

In a medium sauté pan set over low heat, sauté the onion in the coconut oil and the broth until it is translucent. Add the garlic, ginger, crushed red pepper, and broccoli, and sauté the mixture 3 to 4 more minutes. Add the eggs, and using a heat-resistant spatula, gently and continually push the eggs into the center of the pan until everything is cooked through. Slide the scramble onto a serving plate and serve.

Energy Accessory Ideas:

Whole grain: serve the scramble over ½ cup cooked brown rice

or

Starchy vegetable: serve the scramble over ½ cup each shredded raw carrots and chopped jicama

or

Fruit: serve with 1 cup fresh fruit

or

Pulse: serve with ½ cup cooked adzuki beans

Roasted Vegetable Omelet

. . . .

Lean protein: **½ cup organic egg whites or 1 whole organic egg and 3 whites, whisked**

Vegetable: **¼ cup each diced eggplant, diced red onion, and halved grape tomatoes (about 8); ½ cup baby spinach leaves**

Plant-based fat: **1 tablespoon extra-virgin olive oil**

Seasoning suggestion: **½ teaspoon minced garlic, 1 teaspoon balsamic vinegar, ½ teaspoon salt-free Italian seasoning**

Preheat the oven to 350°F. In a medium bowl, combine the olive oil with the eggplant, onion, and tomatoes and toss gently to coat everything. Transfer the vegetables to a baking sheet and roast them for about 10 minutes, until they are very tender. Meanwhile, spray a small sauté pan with an olive oil–based nonstick spray and place the pan over low heat. Whisk the garlic and Italian seasoning into the eggs and pour them into the pan. Allow the eggs to just set, top them with the spinach, and then carefully fold one side over onto the other. Slide the omelet from the pan, top it with the roasted vegetables, and drizzle it with the balsamic vinegar.

Energy Accessory Ideas:

Whole grain: serve the omelet over ½ cup cooked quinoa

or

Starchy vegetable: serve with ½ cup Oven-Roasted Sweet Potato "Fries" (see page 175) or Baked Purple Sweet Potato (see page 174)

or

Fruit: serve with 1 cup fresh fruit

or

Pulse: roast ½ cup chickpeas along with the vegetables

Chilled Sesame Egg Salad—Quick!, Make Ahead, Take It with You

Lean protein: **1 whole hard-boiled organic egg and 3 hard-boiled organic egg whites, chopped**

Vegetable: **½ cup finely chopped kale, ¼ cup minced red onion, ¼ cup halved grape tomatoes**

Plant-based fat: **2 tablespoons tahini**

Seasoning suggestion: **1 teaspoon fresh-squeezed lemon juice, ⅛ teaspoon cayenne pepper, ⅛ teaspoon ground cumin, ½ teaspoon minced garlic**

In a medium bowl, whisk together the lemon juice, cayenne, cumin, garlic, tahini, and 1 tablespoon of water. Add the kale, onion, and tomatoes, and toss to coat everything thoroughly. Gently fold in the eggs and refrigerate the salad for at least 30 minutes before serving.

Energy Accessory Ideas:

Whole grain: spread the salad onto 1 serving (according to the package) 100 percent whole-grain crackers or 1 slice 100 percent whole-grain bread

or

Starchy vegetable: serve with 1 cup raw carrot sticks

or

Fruit: serve with 1 cup fresh fruit

or

Pulse: add ½ cup cooked lentils to the mixture with the eggs

Spinach Walnut Salad—Quick!

Lean protein: **1 whole hard-boiled organic egg and 3 hard-boiled organic egg whites, chopped**

Vegetable: **1 cup baby spinach leaves, ¼ cup sliced white button mushrooms, 2 tablespoons minced red onion**

Plant-based fat: **2 tablespoons chopped walnuts**

Seasoning suggestion: **2 teaspoons Dijon mustard, 2 teaspoons water, 1 teaspoon fresh-squeezed lemon juice, ½ teaspoon minced garlic, ⅛ teaspoon cumin**

In a medium bowl, whisk together the mustard, water, lemon juice, garlic, and cumin. Add the spinach and toss to coat the leaves thoroughly. Transfer the greens to a salad bowl and top them with the mushrooms, onion, egg, and walnuts.

Energy Accessory Ideas:

Whole grain: add ½ cup chilled cooked wild rice to the salad

or

Starchy vegetable: add ½ cup cubed oven-roasted, skin-on red potatoes, warm or
chilled, or Baked Purple Sweet Potato (see page 174) to the salad

or

Fruit: serve with 1 cup fresh fruit

or

Pulse: add ½ cup cooked lentils to the salad

Southwest Egg Salad—*Quick!, Make Ahead, Take It with You*

···

Lean protein: **1 whole hard-boiled organic egg and 3 hard-boiled organic egg
whites, chopped**

Vegetable: **¼ cup quartered grape tomatoes (about 8), 2 tablespoons finely
minced red onion, 3 large outer leaves romaine lettuce**

Plant-based fat: **¼ medium avocado, diced**

Seasoning suggestion: **1 teaspoon chopped fresh cilantro, 1 teaspoon fresh-
squeezed lime juice, 1 small jalapeño (or 1 teaspoon minced), ¹⁄₁₆ teaspoon
black pepper**

In a small bowl, lightly mash the avocado and fold in the cilantro, lime juice, jalapeño,
and pepper. Add the egg and toss to coat everything thoroughly. Spoon the salad
into the romaine leaves, garnish with the tomatoes and onion, and serve.

Energy Accessory Ideas:

Whole grain: sprinkle the filled romaine leaves with ½ cup oven-roasted organic corn

or

Starchy vegetable: serve with ½ cup Oven-Roasted Sweet Potato "Fries" (see
page 175)

or

Fruit: serve with 1 cup fresh fruit

or

Pulse: sprinkle the filled romaine leaves with ½ cup cooked black beans

Savory Veggie Quiche—*Make Ahead, Take It with You*

···

Lean protein: **½ cup organic egg whites or 1 whole organic egg and 3 whites,
whisked**

Vegetable: **¼ cup minced yellow onion, ¼ cup low-sodium organic vegetable
broth, ¼ cup small broccoli florets, ¼ cup chopped white button mushrooms;
½ cup baby spinach leaves**

Plant-based fat: **1 tablespoon extra-virgin coconut oil**
Seasoning suggestion: **½ teaspoon minced garlic, ½ teaspoon salt-free Italian seasoning, ¹⁄₁₆ teaspoon cracked black pepper, ¹⁄₁₆ teaspoon cayenne pepper**

Preheat the oven to 350°F. In a medium sauté pan set over low heat, sauté the onion in the coconut oil and the broth until it is translucent. Add the broccoli, mushrooms, spinach, garlic, Italian seasoning, black pepper, and cayenne, and sauté the mixture 3 or 4 more minutes. Spoon it into a quiche pan, cover it with the eggs, stir it to distribute the vegetables evenly throughout the eggs, and bake the quiche 45 minutes, or until a knife inserted into the center comes out clean.

Energy Accessory Ideas:

Whole grain: add ½ cup cooked quinoa to the quiche

or

Starchy vegetable: serve with ½ cup Oven-Roasted Sweet Potato "Fries" (see page 175) or Baked Purple Sweet Potato (see page 174)

or

Fruit: serve with 1 cup fresh fruit

or

Pulse: add ½ cup cooked lentils or cannellini beans to the quiche

Eggs on the Go—*Quick!, Make Ahead, Take It with You*

Lean protein: **1 whole hard-boiled organic egg and 3 hard-boiled organic egg whites, chopped**
Vegetable: **½ cup each grape tomatoes and green or red bell pepper strips, or 1 cup On-the-Go slaw (see page 175)**
Plant-based fat: **2 tablespoons whole almonds or 10 Mediterranean olives**

Pack all the ingredients into a container and put it in a stay-cold portable sack. (If you pack the slaw, remember to bring a fork!)

Energy Accessory Ideas:

Whole grain: 1 serving (according to the package) 100 percent whole-grain crackers or 3 cups Oil-Free Popped Popcorn (see page 175)

or

Starchy vegetable: 1 cup raw carrot sticks

or

Fruit: 1 cup fresh fruit

or

Pulse: ½ cup Oven-Roasted Chickpeas (see page 175), or omit the almonds or the olives and use hummus as a dip for the raw veggies

• •

WHAT ABOUT DISHES THAT START WITH ENERGY ACCESSORIES, LIKE FRUIT SMOOTHIES AND OATMEAL?

I created each recipe in this chapter by combining the three diet wardrobe staples (lean protein plus veggies plus plant-based fat), along with suggestions for energy accessories that pair well with the trio. But if you love dishes that start with an energy accessory, like fruit, oats, or cereal, you can use the wardrobe design strategy in chapter 3 to build your own meals. All you need to do is work backward. For example, if you want to make oatmeal or a fruit smoothie, use the portion sizes laid out in chapter 3, and pair the oats or fruit with lean protein, veggies, and plant-based fat. The Almond Oatmeal and the Strawberry Peanut Butter Smoothie (recipes follow) show how.

• •

Almond Oatmeal
• •

Lean protein: **¼ cup vanilla-flavored pea protein powder**
Vegetable: **½ cup 100 percent vegetable juice**
Plant-based fat: **2 tablespoons chopped almonds**
Seasoning suggestion: **ground cinnamon or ginger to taste**
Whole grain/fruit energy accessory: **2 tablespoons old-fashioned rolled oats, ½ cup fresh or frozen (thawed) fruit**

Stir the pea protein powder into the oats. Season the mixture with cinnamon or ginger if desired. Pour ¼ cup of hot water into the oats and stir (do not add cold water and heat in the microwave), adding 1 tablespoon more water at a time as needed until the oatmeal is your desired consistency. Add the fruit, top the oatmeal with the almonds, and enjoy the vegetable juice as a side.

Strawberry Peanut Butter Smoothie

....

Lean protein: **1 single-serving container or ¾ cup nonfat vanilla-flavored organic Greek yogurt**
Vegetable: **1 cup baby spinach leaves**
Plant-based fat: **2 tablespoons natural peanut butter**
Fruit energy accessory: **1 cup frozen strawberries**

In a blender, whip the yogurt, spinach, peanut butter, and strawberries with ½ cup of water and a handful of ice until the mixture is smooth; serve.

Remember that you can also include half portions of two different energy accessories, which means you can enjoy both fruit and oats together. Or, based on your My Energy Needs quiz results (see page 87), you may need two full energy accessory servings at one or more of your meals.

Oh, and if you love smoothies, I hope you'll try the Lemon Mint Avocado Smoothie (page 132) and Green Goddess Smoothie (page 159) recipes in this chapter. Both are fantastic with fruit whipped in as the energy accessory. While creating these recipes, I became obsessed with trying the Lemon Mint Avocado Smoothie with a different fruit each day. My favorites are frozen blueberries, strawberries, papaya and pineapple chunks, and kiwi. I also included a bonus Cherry Chocolate Green Goddess Smoothie recipe I think you'll love (page 160)!

....

REMEMBER, YOU CAN CUSTOMIZE ANY RECIPE WITH TRADE-OUTS!

Just like with your attire, where you can mix and match clothing items to create different outfits. I designed this plan to allow you to do the same. Here are six more ways to enjoy oatmeal and fruit smoothies by taking the same wardrobe design framework.

....

Nut-of-Your-Choice Oatmeal

Lean protein: ¼ cup vanilla-flavored pea protein powder
Vegetable: ½ cup 100 percent vegetable juice
Plant-based fat: 2 tablespoons chopped nuts of your choice (walnuts, cashews, macadamia nuts, hazelnuts)
Seasoning suggestion: cinnamon, ginger, nutmeg, apple pie spice, or other spice of your choice, to taste
Whole grain/fruit energy accessory: 2 tablespoons old-fashioned rolled oats, ½ cup fresh or frozen (thawed) fruit

Stir the pea protein powder into the oats and season the mixture with the spice of your choice. Pour ¼ cup of hot water into the oats and stir (do not add cold water and heat in the microwave), adding 1 more tablespoon of water at a time as needed until the oatmeal is your desired consistency. Add the fruit, top the oatmeal with the nuts, and enjoy the vegetable juice as a side.

Note: You can also omit the pea protein powder and have a single-serving container or ¾ cup nonfat vanilla-flavored organic Greek yogurt on the side with your oatmeal.

Mango Coconut Smoothie

Lean protein: 1 single-serving container or ¾ cup nonfat vanilla-flavored organic Greek yogurt
Vegetable: ½ cup chopped cucumber, ½ cup chopped celery
Plant-based fat: 1 tablespoon extra-virgin coconut oil
Fruit energy accessory: 1 cup frozen mango chunks

Combine the yogurt, cucumber, celery, coconut oil, and mango in a blender with ½ cup of water and a handful of ice, and blend the mixture until it is smooth; serve.

Pineapple Macadamia Nut Smoothie

Lean protein: 1 single-serving container or ¾ cup nonfat vanilla-flavored organic Greek yogurt
Vegetable: ½ cup chopped cucumber, ½ cup chopped celery
Plant-based fat: 2 tablespoons macadamia nut butter
Fruit energy accessory: 1 cup frozen pineapple chunks

Combine the yogurt, cucumber, celery, nut butter, and pineapple in a blender with ½ cup of water and a handful of ice, and blend the mixture until it is smooth; serve.

Apple Walnut Smoothie

....

Lean protein: **1 single-serving container or ¾ cup nonfat vanilla-flavored organic Greek yogurt**
Vegetable: **1 cup baby spinach leaves**
Plant-based fat: **2 tablespoons walnut butter**
Fruit energy accessory: **1 small green apple, skin on, cored and diced**

Combine the yogurt, spinach, walnut butter, and apple in a blender with ½ cup of water and a handful of ice, and blend the mixture until it is smooth; serve.

Blueberry Coconut Smoothie

....

Lean protein: **1 single-serving container or ¾ cup nonfat vanilla-flavored organic Greek yogurt**
Vegetable: **1 cup baby spinach leaves**
Plant-based fat: **1 tablespoon extra-virgin coconut oil**
Fruit energy accessory: **1 cup frozen blueberries**

Combine the yogurt, spinach, coconut oil, and blueberries in a blender with ½ cup of water and a handful of ice, and blend the mixture until it is smooth; serve.

Peach Pecan Smoothie

....

Lean protein: **1 single-serving container or ¾ cup nonfat vanilla-flavored organic Greek yogurt**
Vegetable: **½ cup chopped cucumber, ½ cup chopped celery**
Plant-based fat: **2 tablespoons pecan butter**
Fruit energy accessory: **1 cup frozen peaches**

Combine the yogurt, cucumber, celery, pecan butter, and peaches in a blender with ½ cup of water and a handful of ice, and blend the mixture until it is smooth; serve.

Dairy-Based Meals

•••

WHY YOU WON'T FIND MEALS MADE WITH HARD CHEESES AND FULL-FAT DAIRY

Research has shown that animal-based fats, like full-fat cheeses, are less satiating than plant-based fats. In other words, plant-based fats like avocados and nuts help regulate your appetite and keep your weight under control. Unlike full-fat dairy products, they also help lower your LDL cholesterol, raise your HDL cholesterol, and keep your arteries soft and flexible, reducing your risk of heart attack and stroke. For this reason, I've included only nonfat versions of protein-rich dairy products and paired them with plant-based fats, such as extra-virgin olive and coconut oils, nuts, seeds, and nut butters.

•••

Chilled Pesto Cheesy Salad—Quick!, Make Ahead, Take It with You

•••

Lean protein: **½ cup nonfat organic cottage cheese**
Vegetable: **½ cup shredded zucchini, ¼ cup minced red bell pepper, 2 tablespoons minced red onion**
Plant-based fat: **1 tablespoon basil pesto**

In a medium bowl, stir the pesto into the cottage cheese; add the zucchini, pepper, and onion, and toss. Chill the salad for at least 30 minutes before serving.

Energy Accessory Ideas:
Whole grain: add ½ cup cooked quinoa to the salad
or

Starchy vegetable: add ½ cup cubed oven-roasted, skin-on red potatoes to the salad
or
Fruit: serve with 1 cup fresh fruit
or
Pulse: add ½ cup cooked lentils to the salad

Veggies with Mediterranean Olive Dip—Quick!, Make Ahead, Take It with You

Lean protein: **1 single-serving container or ¾ cup nonfat plain organic Greek yogurt**
Vegetable: **1 small red bell pepper, sliced into strips; ½ cup small broccoli florets**
Plant-based fat: **2 tablespoons green and black olive tapenade**
Seasoning suggestion: **1 teaspoon minced garlic, 1 teaspoon salt-free Italian seasoning, ½ tablespoon balsamic vinegar**

Fold the tapenade, garlic, Italian seasoning, and balsamic vinegar into the yogurt. Serve the mixture as a dip with the veggies.

Energy Accessory Ideas:

Whole grain: serve with 1 serving (according to the package) 100 percent whole-grain crackers, or add ½ cup cooked quinoa to the dip
or
Starchy vegetable: serve with ½ cup Oven-Roasted Sweet Potato "Fries" (see page 175)
or
Fruit: serve with 1 cup fresh fruit
or
Pulse: add ¼ cup unsweetened pea protein powder to the dip

Garlicky Spinach Ricotta Sauté—Quick!, Make Ahead, Take It with You, Freeze & Reheat

Lean protein: **¼ cup nonfat organic ricotta cheese**
Vegetable: **1½ cups chopped baby spinach leaves, ¼ cup minced yellow onion**
Plant-based fat: **1 tablespoon extra-virgin olive oil**
Seasoning suggestion: **1 teaspoon minced garlic, ½ teaspoon salt-free Italian seasoning**

In a medium sauté pan set over low heat, sauté the onion in the olive oil until it is translucent. Add the garlic, Italian seasoning, and spinach, and stir just until the spinach wilts. Add the ricotta, stir the mixture until it is heated through, and serve.

Energy Accessory Ideas:

Whole grain: serve over ½ cup cooked whole-grain penne, spoon onto 1 slice 100 percent whole-grain toast, or add ½ cup cooked wild rice to the sauté with the ricotta

or

Starchy vegetable: serve with ½ cup cubed oven-roasted fingerling potatoes

or

Fruit: serve with 1 cup fresh fruit

or

Pulse: add ½ cup chickpeas to the sauté with the ricotta

Roasted Vegetable Spread—Make Ahead, Take It with You

Lean protein: **1 single serving container or ¾ cup nonfat plain organic Greek yogurt**

Vegetable: **½ cup each diced red bell pepper and diced eggplant; ¼ cup chopped red onion**

Plant-based fat: **1 tablespoon extra-virgin olive oil**

Seasoning suggestion: **1 teaspoon minced garlic, ⅛ teaspoon cayenne pepper, ⅛ teaspoon ground cumin**

Preheat the oven to 400°F. Toss the bell pepper, eggplant, and onion with the olive oil, spread the vegetables on a baking sheet, and roast them for 20 minutes or until they are tender. In a food processor, puree the vegetables with the yogurt, garlic, cayenne, and cumin. Reheat the spread or serve it chilled.

Energy Accessory Ideas:

Whole grain: spread onto 1 serving (according to the package) 100 percent whole-grain crackers

or

Starchy vegetable: serve with 1 cup raw baby carrots or carrot sticks

or

Fruit: serve with 1 cup fresh fruit

or

Pulse: add ¼ cup unsweetened pea protein powder to the puree

Cheesy Cauliflower Casserole—Make Ahead, Take It with You, Freeze & Reheat

Lean protein: **½ cup nonfat organic cottage cheese**

Vegetable: **¼ cup minced yellow onion, 2 tablespoons low-sodium organic vegetable broth, ¾ cup small cauliflower florets**

Plant-based fat: **1 tablespoon extra-virgin coconut oil**

Seasoning suggestion: **1 teaspoon minced garlic, ⅛ teaspoon black pepper, 1 teaspoon salt-free Italian seasoning**

Preheat the oven to 350°F. In a medium sauté pan set over low heat, sauté the onion in the coconut oil and the broth until it is translucent. Add the cauliflower, garlic, and Italian seasoning, and sauté the mixture until the cauliflower is slightly tender. In a small baking dish, combine the cauliflower mixture with the cottage cheese and black pepper. Bake the casserole for 20 minutes.

Energy Accessory Ideas:

Whole grain: add ½ cup cooked wild rice with the cottage cheese before baking

or

Starchy vegetable: add 1 cup cooked spaghetti squash with the cottage cheese before baking

or

Fruit: serve with 1 cup fresh fruit

or

Pulse: add ½ cup cannellini beans or chickpeas with the cottage cheese before baking

Dilled Cucumber Tomato Salad—Quick!, Make Ahead, Take It with You

Lean protein: **1 single-serving container or ¾ cup nonfat plain organic Greek yogurt**

Vegetable: **1 small cucumber, sliced thin; 1 small vine-ripened tomato, sliced thin; ¼ cup minced red onion**

Plant-based fat: **2 tablespoons chopped walnuts**

Seasoning suggestion: **1½ tablespoons chopped fresh dill, 1 teaspoon minced garlic, 1 tablespoon red wine vinegar, ⅛ teaspoon black pepper, 1/16 teaspoon cayenne pepper**

In a medium bowl, combine the yogurt, dill, garlic, vinegar, black pepper, and cayenne. Add the cucumber and tomato, and toss to coat everything. Refrigerate the salad for at least 30 minutes. Garnish it with the red onion and walnuts before serving.

Energy Accessory Ideas:

Whole grain: add ½ cup cooked quinoa to the salad with the yogurt before chilling, or sprinkle the salad with ¼ cup Toasted Quinoa (see page 174) just before serving

or

Starchy vegetable: serve with ½ cup cubed oven-roasted, skin-on red potatoes, warm or chilled

or

Fruit: serve with 1 cup fresh fruit

or

Pulse: add ½ cup black-eyed peas with the yogurt before chilling

Chilled Italian Stuffed Tomatoes—*Quick!, Make Ahead, Take It with You*

Lean protein: **¼ cup nonfat organic ricotta cheese**

Vegetable: **4 small whole vine-ripened tomatoes; ¼ cup finely minced yellow onion; ½ cup chopped kale**

Plant-based fat: **1 tablespoon extra-virgin olive oil**

Seasoning suggestion: **1 teaspoon minced garlic, ½ teaspoon salt-free Italian seasoning, ⅛ teaspoon black pepper**

Slice the stems off the tomatoes, scoop out and discard the seeds, and set the tomatoes aside. In a medium sauté pan set over low heat, sauté the onion in the olive oil until it is translucent. Add the kale, garlic, Italian seasoning, black pepper, and ricotta, and stir to mix well and heat everything through. Stuff the tomatoes with the kale-ricotta mixture, then chill them at least 30 minutes before serving.

Energy Accessory Ideas:

Whole grain: add ½ cup cooked quinoa or wheat berries to the ricotta mixture before stuffing the tomatoes

or

Starchy vegetable: serve with ½ cup oven-baked fingerling potatoes, warm or chilled

or

Fruit: serve with 1 cup fresh fruit

or

Pulse: add ½ cup cannellini beans to the ricotta mixture before stuffing the tomatoes

Lemon Mint Avocado Smoothie—Quick!

Lean protein: **1 single-serving container or ¾ cup nonfat vanilla-flavored organic Greek yogurt**
Vegetable: **1 cup baby spinach leaves**
Plant-based fat: **¼ medium avocado**
Seasoning suggestion: **1 tablespoon fresh-squeezed lemon juice; 2 large fresh mint leaves, chopped**

Combine the yogurt, spinach, avocado, lemon juice, and mint with ½ cup of water and a handful of ice, and blend the mixture until it is smooth.

Energy Accessory Ideas:

Whole grain: add ¼ cup old-fashioned rolled oats to the smoothie
or
Starchy vegetable: add ½ cup 100 percent carrot juice to the smoothie
or
Fruit: add 1 cup frozen fruit, such as pineapple or papaya, and omit the ice
or
Pulse: add ¼ cup unsweetened pea protein powder to the smoothie

Roasted Vegetable "Lasagna"—Make Ahead, Take It with You, Freeze & Reheat

Lean protein: **½ cup nonfat organic cottage cheese**
Vegetable: **1 roma tomato, cut into thin rounds; ½ medium zucchini, sliced into ¼-inch rounds; 1 large whole portobello mushroom cap**
Plant-based fat: **1 tablespoon extra-virgin olive oil**
Seasoning suggestion: **1 teaspoon minced garlic, ½ teaspoon salt-free Italian seasoning, ⅛ teaspoon black pepper, ¹⁄₁₆ teaspoon cayenne pepper**

Preheat the oven to 350°F. Place the tomato and zucchini slices and the mushroom in a single layer on a baking sheet and brush or rub them with the olive oil. Roast the vegetables for 15 minutes. Meanwhile, in a small bowl, fold the garlic, Italian seasoning, black pepper, and cayenne into the cottage cheese. Remove the vegetables from the oven, and on a second baking sheet, layer the vegetables with the cottage cheese mixture: using the mushroom as the base, layer with half the ricotta, then the zucchini, then more ricotta, then the tomatoes. Return the "lasagna" to the oven and cook it for an additional 15 minutes.

Energy Accessory Ideas:

Whole grain: add ½ cup cooked quinoa to the ricotta mixture or serve the "lasagna" with ½ cup cooked 100 percent whole-grain penne
or

Starchy vegetable: serve with 1 cup cooked spaghetti squash or ½ cup Baked Purple
   Sweet Potato (see page 174)

or

Fruit: serve with 1 cup fresh fruit

or

Pulse: serve with ½ cup Oven-Roasted Chickpeas (see page 175)

Cheesy Moroccan Lettuce Cups—Quick!

Lean protein: **½ cup nonfat organic cottage cheese**
Vegetable: **1 small minced roma tomato, 2 tablespoons minced red onion,
   3 or 4 large outer leaves romaine lettuce**
Plant-based fat: **1 tablespoon extra-virgin olive oil**
Seasoning suggestion: **2 teaspoons fresh-squeezed lemon juice; ½ teaspoon
   minced garlic; ⅛ teaspoon ground cumin; and ¹⁄₁₆ teaspoon each ground
   coriander, turmeric, cinnamon, and black pepper**

In a small bowl, whisk together the olive oil, lemon juice, garlic, cumin, coriander,
turmeric, cinnamon, and pepper, and fold in the cottage cheese. Fill the romaine
leaves with the cheese mixture, top each leaf with some of the tomato and onion,
and serve.

Energy Accessory Ideas:
Whole grain: add ½ cup cooked wild rice to the cottage cheese mixture

or

Starchy vegetable: serve with ½ cup cubed oven-roasted, skin-on red potatoes,
   warm or chilled

or

Fruit: serve with 1 cup fresh fruit

or

Pulse: add ½ cup chickpeas to the cottage cheese mixture

Sesame Ricotta Dip—Quick!, Make Ahead, Take It with You

Lean protein: **¼ cup nonfat organic ricotta cheese**
Vegetable: **½ cup raw fresh whole snow peas, ½ cup red bell pepper strips**
Plant-based fat: **2 tablespoons tahini**
Seasoning suggestion: **½ teaspoon minced garlic, 2 teaspoons fresh-squeezed
   lemon juice, ¹⁄₁₆ teaspoon black pepper, ¹⁄₁₆ teaspoon ground cumin**

In a small bowl, whisk together the tahini, garlic, lemon juice, pepper, and cumin, and fold in the ricotta. Serve the dip with the snow peas and bell pepper strips.

Energy Accessory Ideas:

Whole grain: serve with 1 serving (according to the package) 100 percent whole-grain crackers

or

Starchy vegetable: serve with ½ cup Oven-Roasted Sweet Potato "Fries" (see page 175)

or

Fruit: serve with 1 cup fresh fruit

or

Pulse: add ½ cup cooked lentils to the ricotta mixture

Cheesy Savory Stuffed Pepper—*Make Ahead, Take It with You, Freeze & Reheat*

Lean protein: **½ cup nonfat organic cottage cheese**
Vegetable: **1 large whole green bell pepper, ¼ cup minced yellow onion, ¼ cup low-sodium organic vegetable broth, ½ cup finely chopped fresh spinach**
Plant-based fat: **1 tablespoon extra-virgin coconut oil**
Seasoning suggestion: **1 teaspoon minced garlic, ½ teaspoon salt-free Italian seasoning, ⅛ teaspoon crushed red pepper flakes, 1/16 teaspoon black pepper**

Preheat the oven to 350°F. Slice off the top of the bell pepper and reserve it. Remove and discard the seeds and inner membranes, and set aside the pepper. In a medium sauté pan set over low heat, sauté the onion in the coconut oil and the broth until it is translucent. Add the spinach, garlic, Italian seasoning, crushed red pepper, and black pepper, and sauté the mixture for 2 to 3 more minutes. Add the cottage cheese and mix well to heat everything through. Spoon the cottage cheese mixture into the bell pepper, place the top on the pepper, and set it in a small baking dish. Cover the dish with foil and bake for 20 minutes; remove the foil and bake the pepper an additional 10 minutes.

Energy Accessory Ideas:

Whole grain: add ½ cup cooked brown rice to the pan with the cottage cheese

or

Starchy vegetable: serve with 1 cup cooked spaghetti squash

or

Fruit: serve with 1 cup fresh fruit

or

Pulse: add ½ cup cannellini beans to the pan with the cottage cheese

Dairy on the Go—Quick!, Make Ahead, Take It with You
....

Lean protein: ½ cup nonfat organic cottage cheese
Vegetable: 1 cup sliced raw veggies, such as celery sticks, sliced zucchini, and
    sliced bell peppers, or On-the-Go slaw (see page 175)
Plant-based fat: 10 herbed Mediterranean olives

Add the olives to the cottage cheese to use as a dip with the veggies. Pack all the
vegetables and the dip in containers and put them in a stay-cold portable sack. (If
you pack the slaw, remember to bring a fork!)

Energy Accessory Ideas:
Whole grain: serve with 1 serving (according to the package) 100 percent whole-grain
    crackers or 3 cups Oil-Free Popped Popcorn (see page 175)
or
Starchy vegetable: add 1 cup baby carrots to the vegetable assortment
or
Fruit: serve with 1 cup fresh fruit
or
Pulse: serve with ½ cup Oven-Roasted Chickpeas (see page 175) or omit the olives
    and use hummus as a dip for the raw veggies

If you enjoy chocolate and want to include it in your meal plan, remember
that you can use the wardrobe design strategy in chapter 3 to build your
own DIY meals—the Chocolate Raspberry Parfait below, for example.

Chocolate Raspberry Parfait
....

Lean protein: 1 single-serving container or ¾ cup nonfat vanilla-flavored organic
    Greek yogurt
Vegetable: ½ cup 100 percent vegetable juice
Plant-based fat: 1 ounce dark chocolate (at least 70 percent cacao), chopped
Seasoning suggestion: ¼ teaspoon grated fresh ginger or ground cinnamon
Fruit energy accessory: 1 cup fresh or thawed frozen raspberries

Fold the ginger or cinnamon into the yogurt, then layer it with the berries in a
parfait glass. Top with the chocolate. (Down your veggie juice before diving in.)

Here are five more fruit parfait options (with and without dark chocolate).

Walnut Pear Parfait
....

Lean protein: **1 single-serving container or ¾ cup nonfat vanilla-flavored organic Greek yogurt**
Vegetable: **½ cup 100 percent vegetable juice**
Plant-based fat: **2 tablespoons chopped walnuts**
Seasoning suggestion: **dash of apple pie spice**
Fruit energy accessory: **1 unpeeled pear, diced**

Fold the apple pie spice into the yogurt, then layer it in a parfait glass with the pear and walnuts. [Down your veggie juice before diving in.]

Citrus Sunflower Parfait
....

Lean protein: **1 single-serving container or ¾ cup nonfat vanilla-flavored organic Greek yogurt**
Vegetable: **½ cup 100 percent vegetable juice**
Plant-based fat: **2 tablespoons sunflower seeds**
Seasoning suggestion: **¼ teaspoon grated fresh ginger**
Fruit energy accessory: **1 cup diced citrus, such as blood orange, pink grapefruit, or tangerine**

Fold the ginger into the yogurt, then layer it in a parfait glass with the citrus and sunflower seeds. [Down your veggie juice before diving in.]

Blueberry Mint Dark Chocolate Parfait
....

Lean protein: **1 single-serving container or ¾ cup nonfat vanilla-flavored organic Greek yogurt**
Vegetable: **½ cup 100 percent vegetable juice**
Plant-based fat: **1 ounce dark chocolate (at least 70 percent cacao), chopped**
Seasoning suggestion: **3 or 4 fresh mint leaves, chopped**
Fruit energy accessory: **1 cup fresh or thawed frozen blueberries**

Fold the mint into the yogurt, then layer it in a parfait glass with the blueberries and dark chocolate chunks. [Down your veggie juice before diving in.]

Pineapple Ginger Coconut Parfait

Lean protein: **1 single-serving container or ¾ cup nonfat vanilla-flavored organic Greek yogurt**
Vegetable: **½ cup 100 percent vegetable juice**
Plant-based fat: **2 tablespoons unsweetened shredded or flaked coconut**
Seasoning suggestion: **¼ teaspoon grated fresh ginger**
Fruit energy accessory: **1 cup fresh or thawed frozen diced pineapple**

Fold the ginger into the yogurt, then layer it in a parfait glass with the pineapple and coconut. [Down your veggie juice before diving in.]

Banana Chia Chocolate Parfait

Lean protein: **1 single-serving container or ¾ cup nonfat vanilla-flavored organic Greek yogurt**
Vegetable: **½ cup 100 percent vegetable juice**
Plant-based fat: **1 tablespoon chia seeds; ½ ounce dark chocolate (at least 70 percent cacao), chopped**
Fruit energy accessory: **½ cup sliced fresh banana**

Fold the chia seeds into the yogurt, then chill the mixture in the refrigerator for about 15 minutes. In a parfait glass, layer the yogurt mixture with the banana and chocolate chunks. [Down your veggie juice before diving in.]

Poultry-Based Meals

Broccoli Cashew Chicken Stir-Fry—Make Ahead, Freeze & Reheat

Lean protein: **3 ounces cooked boneless skinless chicken breast, chopped**
Vegetable: **¼ cup minced yellow onion, ¼ cup low-sodium organic vegetable broth, ¾ cup small broccoli florets**
Plant-based fat: **2 tablespoons chopped cashews**
Seasoning suggestion: **1 teaspoon minced garlic, ¼ teaspoon grated fresh ginger, ⅛ teaspoon crushed red pepper flakes, ⅛ teaspoon black pepper**

In a medium sauté pan set over high heat, sauté the onion in the broth until it is translucent. Add the broccoli, garlic, ginger, crushed red pepper, black pepper, and 1 tablespoon of water, and sauté the mixture until the broccoli is slightly tender. Add the chicken, heat it through, and transfer the stir-fry to a serving dish. Garnish it with the cashews and serve.

Energy Accessory Ideas:
Whole grain: serve over ½ cup cooked brown rice
or
Starchy vegetable: serve over 1 cup cooked spaghetti squash
or
Fruit: add 1 cup fresh fruit, such as seedless orange slices, to the stir-fry
or
Pulse: add ½ cup black-eyed peas with the broccoli

Simple Chicken Cacciatore—Make Ahead, Freeze & Reheat

Lean protein: **3 ounces cooked boneless skinless chicken breast, shredded**
Vegetable: **¼ cup minced yellow onion, ¼ cup low-sodium organic vegetable broth, ¾ cup halved grape tomatoes (about 16), ¼ cup minced green bell pepper**
Plant-based fat: **1 tablespoon extra-virgin olive oil**
Seasoning suggestion: **1 teaspoon minced garlic, 1 teaspoon salt-free Italian seasoning, ⅛ teaspoon black pepper, 2 teaspoons fresh-squeezed lemon juice**

In a medium sauté pan set over low heat, sauté the onion in the olive oil and the broth until it is translucent. Add the tomatoes, bell pepper, garlic, Italian seasoning, black pepper, and lemon juice, and sauté the mixture until the tomatoes are tender. Add the chicken and heat it through; serve.

Energy Accessory Ideas:
Whole grain: serve with ½ cup cooked whole-grain penne
or
Starchy vegetable: serve over 1 cup cooked spaghetti squash
or
Fruit: serve with 1 cup fresh fruit
or
Pulse: add ½ cup cannellini beans with the tomatoes

Turkey and Spinach Stuffed Pepper—Make Ahead, Freeze & Reheat
....

Lean protein: **3 ounces cooked ground turkey (at least 93 percent lean)**
Vegetable: **1 large whole red bell pepper, ¼ cup minced yellow onion, ¼ cup low-sodium organic vegetable broth, ½ cup finely chopped baby spinach leaves**
Plant-based fat: **2 tablespoons sunflower seeds**
Seasoning suggestion: **1 teaspoon minced garlic, 1 teaspoon salt-free Italian seasoning, ⅛ teaspoon crushed red pepper flakes, ⅛ teaspoon black pepper**

Preheat the oven to 350°F. Slice off the top of the bell pepper and reserve it. Remove and discard the seeds and inner membranes, and set aside the pepper. In a medium sauté pan set over low heat, sauté the onion in the broth until it is translucent. Add the spinach, garlic, Italian seasoning, crushed red pepper, and black pepper, and sauté the mixture 2 to 3 more minutes. Add the turkey and heat it through, then stir in the sunflower seeds. Spoon the turkey mixture into the bell pepper, place the top on the pepper, and set it in a small baking dish. Cover the dish with foil, and bake the pepper for 20 minutes; remove the foil and bake the pepper an additional 10 minutes.

Energy Accessory Ideas:
Whole grain: add ½ cup cooked quinoa to the turkey mixture
or
Starchy vegetable: serve with 1 cup cooked spaghetti squash or ½ cup Baked Purple Sweet Potato [see page 174]
or
Fruit: serve with 1 cup fresh fruit
or
Pulse: add ½ cup cooked lentils to the turkey mixture

Chilled Chicken Dijon Salad—Quick!, Make Ahead, Take It with You

....

Lean protein: **3 ounces cooked boneless skinless chicken breast, diced**
Vegetable: **1 cup chopped baby spinach leaves, ¼ cup minced red onion,
    ¼ cup minced red bell pepper**
Plant-based fat: **1 tablespoon extra-virgin olive oil**
Seasoning suggestion: **2 teaspoons Dijon mustard, 1 teaspoon fresh-squeezed
    lemon juice, ½ teaspoon minced garlic, 1 teaspoon salt-free Italian seasoning**

In a small bowl, whisk together the olive oil, mustard, lemon juice, garlic, and Italian seasoning. Add the spinach, onion, and bell pepper, and toss to coat everything. Chill the salad for at least 30 minutes, then top it with the chicken and serve.

Energy Accessory Ideas:

Whole grain: mix ½ cup cooked wild rice into the salad or serve open faced on 1 slice
    100 percent whole-grain bread
or
Starchy vegetable: mix in ½ cup cubed skin-on, oven-roasted red potatoes
or
Fruit: serve with 1 cup fresh fruit
or
Pulse: add ½ cup fava beans to the salad

Southwest Turkey Cilantro Primavera—Quick!

....

Lean protein: **3 ounces cooked ground turkey (at least 93 percent lean)**
Vegetable: **¼ cup minced yellow onion, ¼ cup low-sodium organic vegetable
    broth, ½ cup minced red bell pepper, ¼ cup sliced white button mushrooms**
Plant-based fat: **¼ ripe avocado, diced**
Seasoning suggestion: **½ teaspoon minced garlic, 1 teaspoon fresh-squeezed
    lime juice, 1 tablespoon minced fresh cilantro, ⅛ teaspoon cayenne pepper,
    ⅛ teaspoon black pepper**

In a medium sauté pan set over low heat, sauté the onion in the broth until it is translucent. Add the bell pepper, mushrooms, garlic, lime juice, cilantro, cayenne, and black pepper, and sauté the mixture until the peppers are tender. Add the turkey, heat it through, and transfer everything to a plate. Top it with the avocado just before serving.

Energy Accessory Ideas:

Whole grain: serve over ½ cup oven-roasted or heated frozen organic corn
or

Starchy vegetable: serve over 1 cup cooked spaghetti squash

or

Fruit: serve with 1 cup fresh fruit

or

Pulse: add ½ cup black beans to the sauté with the turkey

Savory Turkey Stuffed Zucchini—Make Ahead, Freeze & Reheat

Lean protein: **3 ounces cooked ground turkey (at least 93 percent lean)**
Vegetable: **1 large whole zucchini, ¼ cup minced red onion, ¼ cup low-sodium organic vegetable broth**
Plant-based fat: **2 tablespoons sunflower seeds**
Seasoning suggestion: **1 teaspoon minced garlic, 1 teaspoon salt-free Italian seasoning, ⅛ teaspoon ground cumin**

Preheat the oven to 350°F. Trim the stems from the zucchini. Slice it lengthwise, scoop out the flesh, and chop the flesh finely. Set aside the shells and the chopped flesh. In a medium sauté pan set over low heat, sauté the onion in the broth until it is translucent. Add the garlic, Italian seasoning, cumin, and zucchini flesh, and sauté the mixture 2 or 3 more minutes. Add the turkey and sunflower seeds, and heat everything through. Spoon the turkey mixture into the zucchini shells, then set them in a small baking dish, and bake them for 25 minutes.

Energy Accessory Ideas:

Whole grain: add ½ cup quinoa to the turkey mixture or sprinkle the dish with
 ¼ cup Toasted Quinoa (see page 174)

or

Starchy vegetable: serve over a bed of ½ cup oven-roasted or heated frozen
 organic corn

or

Fruit: serve with 1 cup fresh fruit

or

Pulse: serve with a side of ½ cup Oven-Roasted Chickpeas (see page 175)

California Chicken Salad—Quick!

Lean protein: **3 ounces cooked boneless skinless chicken breast, cubed**
Vegetable: **1 cup mixed greens, 1 small sliced vine-ripened tomato,
 ¼ cup minced red onion**
Plant-based fat: **¼ ripe avocado**

Seasoning suggestion: **½ teaspoon minced garlic, 1 tablespoon apple cider
vinegar, 1 tablespoon fresh-squeezed lemon juice, 1 tablespoon chopped
fresh basil, ⅛ teaspoon black pepper**

In a food processor, puree the avocado with the garlic, vinegar, lemon juice, basil,
pepper, and 1 tablespoon of water until the dressing is smooth. Transfer it to a bowl,
add the salad greens, and toss to coat all the leaves. Top the salad with the chicken,
tomato, and onion.

Energy Accessory Ideas:

Whole grain: sprinkle the salad with ½ cup cooked quinoa
or
Starchy vegetable: serve with ½ cup Oven-Roasted Sweet Potato "Fries" (see page 175)
or
Fruit: serve with 1 cup fresh fruit
or
Pulse: add ½ cup chilled green peas to the salad

Turkey and Veggie "Chili"—*Make Ahead, Freeze & Reheat*

Lean protein: **3 ounces cooked ground turkey (at least 93 percent lean)**
Vegetable: **¼ cup each minced yellow onion, zucchini, kale, and green bell
pepper; 1 medium vine ripened tomato, diced; ½ cup low-sodium organic
vegetable broth**
Plant-based fat: **¼ ripe avocado**
Seasoning suggestion: **1 teaspoon minced garlic, 1 tablespoon chopped fresh
cilantro, ⅛ teaspoon cayenne pepper, ⅛ teaspoon black pepper**

In a small sauté pan over medium heat, sauté the onion in 2 tablespoons of the
broth until it is translucent. Add the zucchini, kale, and bell pepper and the remaining
broth, and sauté the vegetables for another 2 to 3 minutes. Add the tomato, garlic,
cilantro, cayenne, and black pepper. Raise the heat to high and bring the mixture to
a boil, then immediately reduce the heat to low and simmer it for 10 to 12 minutes,
stirring occasionally. Stir in the turkey and heat it through. Garnish the 'chili" with the
avocado and serve.

Energy Accessory Ideas:

Whole grain: add ½ cup cooked brown rice or ½ cup roasted or frozen organic corn
with the turkey
or
Starchy vegetable: serve over 1 cup cooked spaghetti squash
or
Fruit: serve with 1 cup fresh fruit
or
Pulse: add ½ cup pinto or black beans with the turkey

Gingery Chicken and Veggie Almond Satay—Quick!, Make Ahead, Freeze & Reheat

Lean protein: **3 ounces cooked boneless skinless chicken breast, cubed**

Vegetable: **¼ cup minced yellow onion, ¼ cup low-sodium organic vegetable broth, ½ cup chopped kale, ¼ cup shredded purple cabbage, ¼ cup minced red bell pepper**

Plant-based fat: **2 tablespoons almond butter**

Seasoning suggestion: **1 teaspoon minced garlic, ¼ teaspoon grated fresh ginger, ⅛ teaspoon ground turmeric, ⅛ teaspoon crushed red pepper flakes**

In a medium sauté pan set over low heat, sauté the onion in the broth until it is translucent. Add the kale, cabbage, and bell pepper, and sauté the vegetables 2 to 3 more minutes. Add the garlic, ginger, turmeric, crushed red pepper, almond butter, and 2 tablespoons of water, and stir until the mixture is well combined. Add the chicken and heat it through; serve.

Energy Accessory Ideas:

Whole grain: serve over ½ cup cooked 100 percent whole-grain buckwheat soba noodles

or

Starchy vegetable: serve over ½ cup each shredded raw carrots and jicama

or

Fruit: serve with 1 cup fresh fruit

or

Pulse: add ½ cup black-eyed peas to the sauté with the spices and almond butter

Fiery Southwest Chicken—Quick!

Lean protein: **3 ounces cooked boneless skinless chicken breast**

Vegetable: **½ cup quartered grape tomatoes (about 16); ¼ cup each minced yellow bell pepper and minced white onion; ¼ cup chopped baby spinach leaves**

Plant-based fat: **¼ ripe avocado, diced**

Seasoning suggestion: **½ teaspoon minced garlic, 1/16 teaspoon cayenne pepper, 1 tablespoon minced fresh cilantro, 1 teaspoon minced jalapeño, 2 tablespoons fresh-squeezed lime juice**

In a medium bowl, toss together the tomatoes, bell pepper, onion, spinach, garlic, cayenne, cilantro, jalapeño, and lime juice. Put the chicken on a plate, top it with the dressed vegetables, garnish it with the avocado, and serve.

Energy Accessory Ideas:

Whole grain: serve over ½ cup oven-roasted or heated frozen organic corn

or

Starchy vegetable: serve with ½ cup Oven-Roasted Sweet Potato "Fries" (see page
   175) or Baked Purple Sweet Potato (see page 174)
or
Fruit: serve with 1 cup fresh fruit
or
Pulse: serve with ½ cup black beans

Chicken and Super Greens Soup—*Make Ahead, Freeze & Reheat*

Lean protein: **3 ounces cooked boneless skinless chicken breast, minced**
Vegetable: **¼ cup minced yellow onion, ½ cup low-sodium organic vegetable
   broth, ½ cup small broccoli florets, ½ cup chopped kale**
Plant-based fat: **1 tablespoon extra-virgin olive oil**
Seasoning suggestion: **1 teaspoon minced garlic, 1 teaspoon salt-free Italian
   seasoning, ¹⁄₁₆ teaspoon black pepper, ⅛ teaspoon crushed red pepper flakes,
   1 teaspoon fresh dill**

In a medium saucepan set over low heat, sauté the onion in the olive oil and
2 tablespoons of the broth until it is translucent. Add the remaining broth, broccoli,
and kale, and sauté for 2 to 3 minutes more. Stir in the garlic, Italian seasoning, black
pepper, crushed red pepper, and half of the dill. Add ½ cup of water, raise the heat to
high, and bring the soup to a boil, then immediately reduce the heat to medium-low
and simmer, stirring occasionally, for about 10 minutes. Stir in the chicken and the
remaining dill, and heat the chicken through; serve.

Energy Accessory Ideas:

Whole grain: add ½ cup cooked brown rice or organic corn to the finished soup
or
Starchy vegetable: add ½ cup oven-roasted, skin-on red potatoes to the finished soup
or
Fruit: serve with 1 cup fresh fruit
or
Pulse: add ½ cup lima beans to the soup

Ginger Turkey Avocado Lettuce Cups—*Quick!*

Lean protein: **3 ounces cooked ground turkey (at least 93 percent lean)**
Vegetable: **¼ cup minced red bell pepper, ¼ cup shredded purple cabbage,
   3 to 4 large outer leaves romaine lettuce**

Plant-based fat: **¼ ripe avocado**

Seasoning suggestion: **¼ teaspoon grated fresh ginger, ½ teaspoon minced garlic, 1 tablespoon apple cider vinegar, 1 tablespoon fresh-squeezed lemon juice, 1 tablespoon chopped fresh basil, ⅛ teaspoon black pepper**

In a food processor, puree the avocado with the ginger, garlic, vinegar, lemon juice, basil, and pepper until the mixture is smooth, adding a little water to thin it if needed. Transfer it to a bowl, add the turkey, and toss to coat everything. Fill the romaine leaves with the turkey mixture and top each leaf with some of the bell pepper and cabbage.

Energy Accessory Ideas:

Whole grain: add ½ cup cooked quinoa to the lettuce cups before filling them with turkey or top the lettuce cups with ¼ cup Toasted Quinoa (see page 174)

or

Starchy vegetable: serve with ½ cup Oven-Roasted Sweet Potato "Fries" (see page 175) or Baked Purple Sweet Potato (see page 174)

or

Fruit: serve with 1 cup fresh fruit

or

Pulse: add ½ cup chickpeas to the lettuce cups with the turkey

Chilled Turkey Pesto Salad—*Quick!, Make Ahead, Take It with You*

Lean protein: **3 ounces cooked boneless skinless turkey breast, diced**

Vegetable: **¼ cup minced red onion; ¼ cup diced cucumber; ¼ cup minced red bell pepper; 1 roma tomato, diced**

Plant-based fat: **1 tablespoon basil pesto**

Place the turkey, onion, cucumber, bell pepper, tomato, and pesto in a sealable container. Seal and shake the container to coat the turkey and vegetables with the pesto. Refrigerate the salad for at least 30 minutes before serving.

Energy Accessory Ideas:

Whole grain: serve with 1 serving (according to the package) 100 percent whole-grain crackers

or

Starchy vegetable: serve with ½ cup Oven-Roasted Sweet Potato "Fries" (see page 175) or Baked Purple Sweet Potato (see page 174)

or

Fruit: serve with 1 cup fresh fruit

or

Pulse: add ½ cup cannellini beans to mixture or serve with ½ cup Oven-Roasted Chickpeas (see page 175)

Curried Chicken and Broccoli Stew—Make Ahead, Freeze & Reheat

....

Lean protein: **3 ounces cooked boneless skinless chicken breast, shredded**

Vegetable: **¼ cup minced yellow onion, ½ cup low-sodium organic vegetable broth, 1½ cups small broccoli florets**

Plant-based fat: **1 tablespoon extra-virgin coconut oil**

Seasoning suggestion: **1 teaspoon minced garlic, 1 tablespoon fresh-squeezed lemon juice, ½ teaspoon curry powder, ⅛ teaspoon paprika, ⅛ teaspoon ground cumin, ⅛ teaspoon black pepper**

In a medium saucepan set over low heat, sauté the onion in the coconut oil and 2 tablespoons of the broth until it is translucent. Add the remaining broth, ½ cup of water, the broccoli, garlic, lemon juice, curry powder, paprika, cumin, and black pepper. Raise the heat to high and bring the mixture to a boil, then immediately reduce the heat to medium-low and simmer the stew, stirring occasionally, for about 10 minutes. Add the chicken and heat it through; serve.

Energy Accessory Ideas:

Whole grain: add ½ cup cooked brown rice to the stew with the chicken

or

Starchy vegetable: add ½ cup oven-roasted, skin-on red potatoes to the stew with the chicken

or

Fruit: serve with 1 cup fresh fruit

or

Pulse: add ½ cup chickpeas to the stew with the chicken

Avocado Basil Dijon Chicken

....

Lean protein: **3 ounces cooked boneless skinless chicken breast, diced**

Vegetable: **¾ cup baby spinach leaves; 1 roma tomato, diced; 2 tablespoons minced red onion**

Plant-based fat: **¼ ripe avocado**

Seasoning suggestion: **1 teaspoon Dijon mustard, 1 teaspoon minced garlic,
½ teaspoon apple cider vinegar, ½ tablespoon fresh-squeezed lime juice,
1 tablespoon chopped fresh basil, ⅛ teaspoon black pepper**

In a food processor, puree the avocado with the mustard, garlic, vinegar, lime juice, basil, pepper, and 1 tablespoon of water until the mixture is smooth. Transfer it to a bowl and add the chicken; stir to coat all the pieces. Place the spinach on a plate, top with the chicken, and drizzle all with the avocado sauce. Sprinkle with the tomato and onion; serve.

Energy Accessory Ideas:

Whole grain: serve with ½ cup cooked quinoa

or

Starchy vegetable: place the spinach over 1 cup cooked spaghetti squash or serve with
   ½ cup oven-roasted fingerling potatoes

or

Fruit: serve with 1 cup fresh fruit

or

Pulse: place the spinach over ½ cup steamed lentils

Poultry on the Go—*Quick!, Make Ahead, Take It with You*
....

Lean Protein: **3 ounces cooked boneless skinless chicken breast, sliced into strips**
Vegetable: **1 cup raw veggies, such as celery, ½ cup each grape tomatoes and
   green or red bell pepper strips, or On-the-Go slaw (see page 175)**
Plant-based fat: **10 herbed Mediterranean olives**

Pack the chicken, veggies, and olives in a container and place it in a stay-cold portable sack (if you pack the slaw, remember to bring a fork!).

Energy Accessory Ideas:

Whole grain: serve with 1 serving (according to the package) 100 percent whole-grain
   crackers or 3 cups Oil-Free Popped Popcorn (see page 175)

or

Starchy vegetable: serve with 1 cup raw carrot sticks

or

Fruit: serve with 1 cup fresh fruit

or

Pulse: serve with ½ cup Oven-Roasted Chickpeas (see page 175) or omit the olives
   and use hummus as a dip for the veggies

Seafood-Based Meals

Lime Pepper Salmon Avocado Salad—Quick!, Take It with You

Lean protein: **3 ounces cooked or canned wild salmon**
Vegetable: **1½ cups baby spinach leaves, ¼ cup halved grape tomatoes, 2 tablespoons minced red onion**
Plant-based fat: **¼ ripe avocado**
Seasoning suggestion: **1 teaspoon minced garlic, 2 teaspoons apple cider vinegar, 1 tablespoon fresh-squeezed lime juice, ¼ teaspoon lime zest, 1 tablespoon chopped fresh cilantro, ⅛ teaspoon black pepper**

In a food processor, puree the avocado with the garlic, vinegar, lime juice, zest, cilantro, pepper, and ½ tablespoon of water until the dressing is smooth. Transfer it to a salad bowl, add the spinach, and toss to coat all the leaves. Top the salad with the salmon, tomatoes, and onion.

Energy Accessory Ideas:

Whole grain: add ½ cup oven-roasted or heated frozen organic corn to the salad
or
Starchy vegetable: serve with ½ cup Oven-Roasted Sweet Potato "Fries" (see page 175) or Baked Purple Sweet Potato (see page 174)
or
Fruit: serve with 1 cup fresh fruit
or
Pulse: add ½ cup green peas to the salad

Ginger Cashew Shrimp Satay—Quick!, Make Ahead, Freeze & Reheat

Lean protein: **3 ounces peeled, deveined, and cooked medium shrimp (frozen is fine)**
Vegetable: **¼ cup minced yellow onion, ¼ cup low-sodium organic vegetable broth, ½ cup small broccoli florets, ¼ cup minced red bell pepper, and ¼ cup chopped fresh kale**
Plant-based fat: **2 tablespoons cashew butter**

Seasoning suggestion: **1 teaspoon minced garlic, ¼ teaspoon grated fresh ginger, ⅛ teaspoon ground turmeric, 1/16 teaspoon crushed red pepper flakes**

In a medium sauté pan set over low heat, sauté the onion in the broth until it is translucent. Add the broccoli, bell pepper, and kale, and sauté the vegetables 2 to 3 more minutes. Add the garlic, ginger, turmeric, crushed red pepper, cashew butter, and 2 tablespoons of water, and stir until everything is well combined. Serve the shrimp over the vegetables.

Energy Accessory Ideas:
Whole grain: serve over ½ cup cooked wild rice
or
Starchy vegetable: serve over 1 cup cooked spaghetti squash
or
Fruit: serve with 1 cup fresh fruit
or
Pulse: add ½ cup black-eyed peas to the sauté with the spices and cashew butter

Chilled Tuna Tahini Salad—*Quick!, Make Ahead, Take It with You*

Lean protein: **3 ounces chunk light tuna, canned in water**
Vegetable: **¼ cup each halved grape tomatoes (about 8), baby spinach leaves, diced cucumber, and minced red onion**
Plant-based fat: **2 tablespoons tahini**
Seasoning suggestion: **1 teaspoon fresh-squeezed lemon juice, 1 teaspoon minced garlic, 1/16 teaspoon cayenne pepper, 1/16 teaspoon black pepper, ⅛ teaspoon ground cumin**

In a medium sealable container, whisk together the lemon juice, garlic, cayenne, black pepper, cumin, tahini, and 2 tablespoons of water. Add the tuna, tomatoes, spinach, cucumber, and onion, seal the container, and gently shake it to coat everything thoroughly. Refrigerate the salad at least 30 minutes before serving.

Energy Accessory Ideas:
Whole grain: add ½ cup cooked quinoa to the salad before chilling it or serve the salad with 1 serving (according to the package) 100 percent whole-grain crackers
or
Starchy vegetable: add ½ cup oven-roasted, skin-on red potatoes before chilling the salad
or
Fruit: serve with 1 cup fresh fruit
or
Pulse: add ½ cup lima beans to the salad before chilling it

Salmon with Garlic Rosemary Roasted Vegetables

Lean protein: **3 ounces baked or grilled wild salmon**

Vegetable: **¼ cup each minced green bell pepper, minced red onion, halved grape tomatoes, and quartered white button mushrooms**

Plant-based fat: **1 tablespoon extra-virgin olive oil**

Seasoning suggestion: **1 teaspoon minced garlic, 1 teaspoon minced fresh rosemary**

Preheat the oven to 350°F. In a small bowl, toss the bell pepper, onion, tomatoes, and mushrooms with the olive oil, garlic, and rosemary. Spread the vegetables on a baking sheet and roast them for 25 minutes. Serve them with the salmon.

Energy Accessory Ideas:

Whole grain: serve with ½ cup cooked wild rice

or

Starchy vegetable: serve with ½ cup oven-roasted butternut squash

or

Fruit: serve with 1 cup fresh fruit

or

Pulse: serve on a bed of ½ cup steamed lentils

Garlicky Shrimp Scampi—*Quick!, Make Ahead, Freeze & Reheat*

Lean protein: **3 ounces peeled, deveined, and cooked medium shrimp (frozen is fine)**

Vegetable: **¼ cup minced yellow onion, ¼ cup low-sodium organic vegetable broth, 1 cup fresh whole snow peas, ¼ cup minced red bell pepper**

Plant-based fat: **1 tablespoon extra-virgin olive oil**

Seasoning suggestion: **1 teaspoon minced garlic, ½ tablespoon fresh-squeezed lemon juice, ⅛ teaspoon grated lemon zest, 1 teaspoon chopped fresh flat-leaf parsley or ½ teaspoon dried, ⅛ teaspoon black pepper**

In a medium sauté pan set over low heat, sauté the onion in the olive oil and 2 tablespoons of the broth until the onion is translucent. Add the snow peas, bell pepper, remaining broth, garlic, lemon juice, zest, parsley, and black pepper, and sauté the mixture 4 to 5 more minutes. Add the cooked shrimp to heat everything through; serve.

Energy Accessory Ideas:

Whole grain: serve over ½ cup cooked wild rice

or

Starchy vegetable: serve over 1 cup cooked spaghetti squash

or

Fruit: serve with 1 cup fresh fruit

or

Pulse: add ½ cup cannellini beans with the shrimp to heat through

Basil Balsamic Tuna Salad—Quick!, Make Ahead, Take It with You

Lean protein: **3 ounces chunk light tuna, canned in water**
Vegetable: **1 roma tomato, diced; ¼ cup each minced red onion, minced yellow bell pepper, and shredded zucchini**
Plant-based fat: **1 tablespoon extra-virgin olive oil**
Seasoning suggestion: **1½ tablespoons balsamic vinegar; ½ tablespoon fresh-squeezed lemon juice; 3 fresh basil leaves, chopped; 1 teaspoon minced garlic; ⅛ teaspoon ground celery seed; ¹⁄₁₆ teaspoon black pepper**

In a sealable container, whisk together the olive oil, vinegar, lemon juice, basil, garlic, celery seed, and black pepper. Add the tuna, tomato, onion, bell pepper, and zucchini, seal the container, and gently shake it to coat everything. Refrigerate the salad for at least 30 minutes before serving.

Energy Accessory Ideas:

Whole grain: add ½ cup cooked wild rice to the salad with the tuna or serve the salad with 1 serving (according to the package) 100 percent whole-grain crackers

or

Starchy vegetable: serve with ½ cup Oven-Roasted Sweet Potato "Fries" (see page 175) or Baked Purple Sweet Potato (see page 174)

or

Fruit: serve with 1 cup fresh fruit

or

Pulse: add ½ cup cannellini beans to the salad with the tuna

Cilantro Shrimp Stuffed Tomatoes—Make Ahead, Freeze & Reheat

Lean protein: **3 ounces peeled, deveined, and cooked medium shrimp, minced (frozen is fine)**
Vegetable: **4 whole small vine-ripened tomatoes, ¼ cup finely minced yellow onion, ½ cup chopped baby spinach leaves**
Plant-based fat: **¼ ripe avocado**

Seasoning suggestion: **1 teaspoon minced garlic, 2 teaspoons apple cider vinegar, 1 tablespoon fresh-squeezed lime juice, 1 tablespoon chopped fresh cilantro, ¹⁄₁₆ teaspoon black pepper**

Slice the stems off the tomatoes, scoop out and discard the seeds, and set the tomatoes aside. In a food processor, puree the avocado with the garlic, vinegar, lime juice, cilantro, pepper, and ½ tablespoon of water until the mixture is smooth. Transfer it to a bowl, add the onion, spinach, and shrimp, and toss. Stuff the tomatoes with the mixture (serve any extra on the side), and chill the tomatoes at least 30 minutes before serving.

Energy Accessory Ideas:

Whole grain: before serving, sprinkle the tomatoes with ¼ cup Toasted Quinoa (see page 174)

or

Starchy vegetable: serve with ½ cup oven-baked fingerling potatoes, warm or chilled, or ½ cup Baked Purple Sweet Potato (see page 174)

or

Fruit: serve with 1 cup fresh fruit

or

Pulse: serve with ½ cup Oven-Roasted Chickpeas (see page 175)

Ginger Coconut Sea Scallops—*Quick!*
....

Lean protein: **3 ounces broiled sea scallops**
Vegetable: **¼ cup minced yellow onion, ¼ cup low-sodium organic vegetable broth, 1 cup chopped fresh kale, ¼ cup minced red bell pepper**
Plant-based fat: **1 tablespoon extra-virgin coconut oil**
Seasoning suggestion: **¼ teaspoon grated fresh ginger, 1 teaspoon minced garlic, ¹⁄₁₆ teaspoon ground cinnamon, ⅛ teaspoon ground cumin, 1 fresh lemon wedge**

In a medium sauté pan set over low heat, sauté the onion in the coconut oil and 2 tablespoons of the broth until it is translucent. Add the kale, bell pepper, ginger, garlic, cinnamon, cumin, and the remaining broth, and sauté the mixture 3 to 4 more minutes. Place the vegetables on a plate and top them with the scallops; squeeze fresh lemon over the scallops just before serving.

Energy Accessory Ideas:

Whole grain: serve with ½ cup cooked wild rice

or

Starchy vegetable: serve with 1 cup cooked spaghetti squash

or

Fruit: serve with 1 cup fresh fruit

or

Pulse: add ½ cup chickpeas to sauté with the kale

Simple Tom Yum Shrimp Soup—*Make Ahead, Freeze & Reheat*

Lean protein: **3 ounces peeled, deveined cooked medium shrimp (frozen is fine)**
Vegetable: **¼ cup minced white onion, ½ cup low-sodium organic vegetable broth, ½ cup small broccoli florets, ¼ cup sliced white button mushrooms, ¼ cup halved grape tomatoes (about 8)**
Plant-based fat: **1 tablespoon extra-virgin coconut oil**
Seasoning suggestion: **1 teaspoon minced garlic, 1 tablespoon fresh-squeezed lime juice, 1 finely chopped dried kaffir lime leaf, ½ tablespoon chopped dried lemongrass, ⅛ teaspoon crushed red pepper flakes**

In a medium saucepan set over low heat, sauté the onion in the coconut oil and 2 tablespoons of the broth until it is translucent. Add the remaining broth, broccoli, and mushrooms, and sauté the mixture for 2 to 3 more minutes. Add ½ cup of water and the garlic, lime juice, kaffir lime leaf, lemongrass, and crushed red pepper. Raise the heat to high and bring the soup to a boil, then immediately reduce the heat and simmer it, stirring occasionally, for about 10 minutes. Stir in the tomatoes and shrimp to heat them through, and serve.

Energy Accessory Ideas:

Whole grain: add ½ cup cooked 100 percent whole-grain buckwheat soba noodles to the soup before serving
or
Starchy vegetable: serve with ½ cup Oven-Roasted Sweet Potato "Fries" (see page 175)
or
Fruit: serve with 1 cup fresh fruit
or
Pulse: add ½ cup lima beans to the soup before serving

Curry Lime Shrimp and Cauliflower Stew—*Make Ahead, Freeze & Reheat*

Lean protein: **3 ounces peeled, deveined, and cooked medium shrimp (frozen is fine)**
Vegetable: **¼ cup minced yellow onion, ½ cup low-sodium organic vegetable broth, 1½ cups small cauliflower florets**
Plant-based fat: **1 tablespoon extra-virgin coconut oil**
Seasoning suggestion: **½ teaspoon minced garlic, 1 tablespoon fresh-squeezed lime juice, ¼ teaspoon lime zest, ¼ teaspoon curry powder, ⅛ teaspoon paprika, 1/16 teaspoon black pepper, ⅛ teaspoon cumin**

In a medium saucepan set over low heat, sauté the onion in the coconut oil and 2 tablespoons of the broth until it is translucent. Add the remaining broth, cauliflower, garlic, lime juice, zest, curry powder, paprika, black pepper, cumin, and ½ cup of water. Raise the heat to high and bring the stew to a boil, then immediately reduce the heat to medium-low and simmer it, stirring occasionally, for about 10 minutes. Add the shrimp to heat it through, and serve.

Energy Accessory Ideas:

Whole grain: add ½ cup cooked wild rice to the stew with the shrimp

or

Starchy vegetable: add ½ cup oven-roasted, skin-on red potatoes to the stew with the shrimp

or

Fruit: serve with 1 cup fresh fruit

or

Pulse: add ½ cup chickpeas to the stew with the shrimp

Salmon Avocado "Tacos"—Quick!

Lean protein: **3 ounces cooked or canned wild salmon, cut into 3 pieces**
Vegetable: **½ cup quartered grape tomatoes (about 16); ¼ cup each minced yellow bell pepper and minced white onion; 3 large outer leaves romaine lettuce**
Plant-based fat: **¼ ripe avocado, diced**
Seasoning suggestion: **1 teaspoon minced garlic, 1/16 teaspoon cayenne pepper, 1 tablespoon minced fresh cilantro, 1 teaspoon minced jalapeño, 2 tablespoons fresh-squeezed lime juice**

In a medium bowl, combine the tomatoes, bell pepper, onion, garlic, cayenne, cilantro, jalapeño, and lime juice. Toss the mixture together and let it marinate in the refrigerator. Fill each romaine leaf with a piece of salmon, top each with the vegetable mixture, and garnish them with avocado.

Energy Accessory Ideas:

Whole grain: add ½ cup organic oven-roasted or heated frozen corn to the "tacos"

or

Starchy vegetable: serve with ½ cup Oven-Roasted Sweet Potato "Fries" (see page 175)

or

Fruit: serve with 1 cup fresh fruit

or

Pulse: add ½ cup black beans to the "tacos"

Ginger Mint Shrimp Stir-Fry—*Quick!, Make Ahead, Freeze & Reheat*

Lean protein: **3 ounces peeled, deveined, and cooked medium shrimp (frozen is fine)**

Vegetable: **¼ cup minced yellow onion, ¼ cup low-sodium organic vegetable broth, ¼ cup minced green bell pepper, ¼ cup minced red bell pepper, ¼ cup shredded purple cabbage**

Plant-based fat: **1 tablespoon extra-virgin coconut oil**

Seasoning suggestion: **1 teaspoon minced garlic; ¼ teaspoon grated fresh ginger; 1 tablespoon chopped fresh mint; 1 small fresh Thai chile pepper, minced, or ⅛ teaspoon crushed red pepper flakes**

In a medium sauté pan set over low heat, sauté the onion in the coconut oil and the broth until it is translucent. Add the bell peppers, cabbage, garlic, ginger, mint, and chile or crushed red pepper, and sauté the mixture until the peppers are slightly tender. Add the shrimp, heat it through, and serve.

Energy Accessory Ideas:

Whole grain: serve over ½ cup cooked brown rice

or

Starchy vegetable: serve over 1 cup cooked spaghetti squash

or

Fruit: serve with 1 cup fresh fruit or add seedless orange slices to the stir-fry

or

Pulse: add ½ cup black-eyed peas with the cabbage

Balsamic Tuna and Brussels Sprout Bake

Lean protein: **3 ounces chunk light tuna canned in water**

Vegetable: **¼ cup minced yellow onion, ¼ cup low-sodium organic vegetable broth, 1 cup quartered baby Brussels sprouts, ¼ cup minced red bell pepper**

Plant-based fat: **1 tablespoon extra-virgin olive oil**

Seasoning suggestion: **1 teaspoon minced garlic, 1 teaspoon fresh-squeezed lemon juice, ½ teaspoon salt-free Italian seasoning, 1 tablespoon balsamic vinegar**

Preheat the oven to 350°F. In a medium sauté pan set over low heat, sauté the onion in the olive oil and 2 tablespoons of the broth until it is translucent. Add the remaining broth, Brussels sprouts, bell pepper, garlic, lemon juice, and Italian seasoning, and sauté the mixture for 3 to 4 more minutes. Stir in the tuna to heat it through, then transfer the mixture to a baking dish, drizzle it with the vinegar, and bake it for 20 minutes.

Energy Accessory Ideas:
Whole grain: add ½ cup cooked quinoa to the dish before baking or sprinkle it with
    ¼ cup Toasted Quinoa (see page 174)
or
Starchy vegetable: serve with ½ cup oven-roasted fingerling potatoes or Baked
    Purple Sweet Potato (see page 174)
or
Fruit: serve with 1 cup fresh fruit
or
Pulse: add ½ cup cannellini beans to sauté with the tuna

Mediterranean Cod with Olives—*Quick!*

Lean protein: **3 ounces baked cod**
Vegetable: **¼ cup minced yellow onion; ¼ cup low-sodium organic vegetable
    broth; 1 small vine ripened tomato, diced small; 1½ cups baby spinach leaves**
Plant-based fat: **10 Mediterranean olives, sliced**
Seasoning suggestion: **1 teaspoon minced garlic, ½ teaspoon salt-free Italian
    seasoning, ¹⁄₁₆ teaspoon each black pepper and cayenne pepper**

In a medium sauté pan set over low heat, sauté the onion in 2 tablespoons of the
broth until it is translucent. Add the spinach, remaining broth, tomato, garlic, Italian
seasoning, black pepper, and cayenne, and sauté the vegetables 3 to 4 minutes
more, or until the tomato is tender. Place the spinach mixture on a plate, top it with
the cod and the olives, and serve.

Energy Accessory Ideas:
Whole grain: serve with ½ cup cooked wild rice
or
Starchy vegetable: serve with 1 cup cooked spaghetti squash or ½ cup oven-roasted
    butternut squash
or
Fruit: serve with 1 cup fresh fruit, such as pineapple chunks
or
Pulse: serve with ½ cup lima beans

Chilled Salmon Pesto Salad—*Quick!, Make Ahead, Take It with You*

Lean protein: **3 ounces cooked or canned wild salmon, flaked**
Vegetable: **¼ cup each minced red onion, minced red bell pepper, shredded
    zucchini, and halved grape tomatoes (about 8)**

Plant-based fat: **1 tablespoon basil pesto**

Place the salmon, onion, bell pepper, zucchini, tomatoes, and pesto in a sealable container. Seal the container and shake it to coat the mixture thoroughly. Refrigerate it for at least 30 minutes before serving.

Energy Accessory Ideas:

Whole grain: serve with 1 serving (according to the package) 100 percent whole-grain crackers

or

Starchy vegetable: serve with ½ cup Oven-Roasted Sweet Potato "Fries" (see page 175)

or

Fruit: serve with 1 cup fresh fruit

or

Pulse: add ½ cup cannellini beans to the mixture or serve with ½ cup Oven-Roasted Chickpeas (see page 175)

Seafood on the Go—Quick!, Make Ahead, Take It with You
....

Lean protein: **1 single-serving pouch or can of either chunk light tuna in water or wild salmon**

Vegetable: **½ cup each grape tomatoes and green or red bell pepper strips, or 1 cup On-the-Go Slaw (see page 175)**

Plant-based fat: **10 Mediterranean olives**

Pack the tuna, veggies, and olives in a sealable container, and place the container in a stay-cold portable sack (if you pack the slaw, remember to bring a fork!).

Energy Accessory Ideas:

Whole grain: serve with 1 serving (according to the package) 100 percent whole-grain crackers or 3 cups Oil-Free Popped Popcorn (see page 175)

or

Starchy vegetable: add 1 cup raw carrot sticks

or

Fruit: serve with 1 cup fresh fruit

or

Pulse: serve with ½ cup Oven-Roasted Chickpeas (see page 175) or omit the olives and use hummus as a dip for the raw veggies

Pulse-Based Meals

Moroccan Lentil Soup—Make Ahead, Freeze & Reheat

Lean protein: ½ **cup cooked lentils**

Vegetable: ¼ **cup minced yellow onion; ½ cup low-sodium organic vegetable broth; ½ cup small cauliflower florets; ½ cup baby spinach leaves; 1 roma tomato, diced**

Plant-based fat: **1 tablespoon extra-virgin coconut oil**

Seasoning suggestion: **1 teaspoon minced garlic; 1 teaspoon fresh-squeezed lemon juice; 1 teaspoon salt-free Italian seasoning; ¹⁄₁₆ teaspoon each ground cinnamon, cumin, turmeric, and coriander**

In a medium saucepan set over low heat, sauté the onion in the coconut oil and 2 tablespoons of the broth until it is translucent. Add the remaining broth, cauliflower, garlic, lemon juice, Italian seasoning, cinnamon, cumin, turmeric, and coriander, and sauté the mixture for 3 to 4 more minutes. Stir in ½ cup of water, the spinach, and the tomato. Raise the heat to high and bring the soup to a boil, then immediately reduce the heat to medium-low and simmer the soup about 10 minutes. Add the lentils and heat them through; serve.

Energy Accessory Ideas:

Whole grain: add ½ cup cooked wild rice to the soup with the lentils

or

Starchy vegetable: add ½ cup oven-roasted, skin-on red potatoes with the lentils

or

Fruit: serve with 1 cup fresh fruit

or

Pulse: double the lentil portion or add ½ cup chickpeas with the lentils

Black Bean "Tacos"—Quick!

Lean protein: ½ **cup cooked black beans**

Vegetable: ¼ **cup each minced white onion and green bell pepper, ¼ cup low-sodium organic vegetable broth, ½ cup quartered grape tomatoes (about 16), 3 or 4 large outer leaves romaine lettuce**

Plant-based fat: ¼ **medium avocado**

Seasoning suggestion: **1 teaspoon chopped fresh cilantro, 1 teaspoon fresh-squeezed lime juice, 1 teaspoon minced jalapeño, ¹⁄₁₆ teaspoon cracked black pepper**

In a bowl, lightly mash the avocado with the cilantro, lime juice, jalapeño, and black pepper to make guacamole; chill. In a medium sauté pan set over low heat, sauté the onion and bell pepper in the broth until the onion is translucent. Add the tomatoes and beans, and sauté the mixture another 2 to 3 minutes to heat it through. Fill the romaine leaves with the veggie mixture, garnish each with some guacamole, and serve.

Energy Accessory Ideas:
Whole grain: add ½ cup oven-roasted or heated frozen organic corn to the "tacos"
or
Starchy vegetable: serve with ½ cup Oven-Roasted Sweet Potato "Fries" (see page 175) or Baked Purple Sweet Potato (see page 174)
or
Fruit: serve with 1 cup fresh fruit
or
Pulse: double the black bean portion or add ½ cup pinto beans

Green Goddess Smoothie—Quick!

Lean protein: **¼ cup vanilla-flavored pea protein powder**
Vegetable: **1 cup baby spinach leaves**
Plant-based fat: **¼ ripe avocado**
Seasoning suggestion: **1 tablespoon fresh-squeezed lime juice, ½ teaspoon grated fresh ginger**

Combine the pea protein, spinach, avocado, lime juice, and ginger in a blender with ¾ cup of water and a handful of ice, and blend the mixture until it is smooth; serve.

Energy Accessory Ideas:
Whole grain: add ¼ cup old-fashioned rolled oats to the smoothie
or
Starchy vegetable: add ½ cup 100 percent carrot juice to the smoothie
or
Fruit: add 1 cup fruit of your choice, such as green grapes, a diced unpeeled green apple, or even a nongreen fruit like frozen berries or cherries
or
Pulse: add ½ cup green peas to the smoothie

One ounce of dark chocolate (at least 70 percent cacao) counts as a serving of plant-based fat, and when I was creating these recipes, I really wanted to include a smoothie with chocolate. However, because this really only works with fruit as the energy accessory (which means I needed to select the energy accessory for you rather than giving you options), I decided to include it as a variation of the Green Goddess Smoothie. Are you thinking that chocolate and spinach don't exactly go together? I promise, you won't even know the spinach is there, and you'll savor every sip of this decadent, dessert-like meal! Note: If you eat dairy, you can replace the pea protein powder with a single-serving container (or ¾ cup) of nonfat vanilla-flavored organic Greek yogurt.

Cherry Chocolate Green Goddess Smoothie!

Lean protein: **¼ cup vanilla-flavored pea protein powder**
Vegetable: **1 cup baby spinach leaves**
Plant-based fat: **1 ounce dark chocolate (at least 70 percent cacao), chopped**
Seasoning suggestion: **1 tablespoon fresh-squeezed lime juice, ½ teaspoon grated fresh ginger**
Fruit energy accessory: **1 cup frozen cherries**

In a blender, combine the protein powder, spinach, chocolate, lime juice, ginger, and cherries with ¾ cup of water, and a handful of ice if desired, and blend the mixture until it is smooth; serve.

Lemon Pepper Hummus—Quick!, Make Ahead, Take It with You

Lean protein: **½ cup cooked chickpeas**
Vegetable: **½ cup small broccoli florets, ½ cup grape tomatoes**
Plant-based fat: **2 tablespoons tahini**
Seasoning suggestion: **1 teaspoon minced garlic; 1 tablespoon fresh-squeezed lemon juice; ¼ teaspoon fresh lemon zest; 1/16 teaspoon each cayenne pepper, black pepper, and cumin**

In a blender or food processor, combine the chickpeas, tahini, garlic, lemon juice, zest, cayenne, black pepper, cumin, and 2 tablespoons of water, and blend the mixture until it is smooth. Serve the hummus with the raw veggies.

Energy Accessory Ideas:

Whole grain: serve with 1 serving (according to the package) 100 percent whole-grain crackers

or

Starchy vegetable: serve with 1 cup baby carrots or carrot sticks

or

Fruit: serve with 1 cup fresh fruit

or

Pulse: fold ½ cup Oven-Roasted Chickpeas (see page 175) into the hummus

Chilled Basil Balsamic Lentil Salad—Quick!, Make Ahead, Take It with You

Lean protein: **½ cup cooked lentils**

Vegetable: **¼ cup each minced red onion, minced cucumber, minced red bell pepper, and halved grape tomatoes (about 8)**

Plant-based fat: **1 tablespoon extra-virgin olive oil**

Seasoning suggestion: **2 tablespoons balsamic vinegar, ½ teaspoon minced garlic, ½ teaspoon salt-free Italian seasoning, 3 chopped fresh basil leaves**

Place all the ingredients in a sealable container. Seal the container and gently shake it to coat everything thoroughly. Refrigerate the salad for at least 30 minutes before serving.

Energy Accessory Ideas:

Whole grain: add ½ cup cooked quinoa to the salad before refrigerating

or

Starchy vegetable: add ½ cup oven-roasted, skin-on red potatoes to the salad before refrigerating

or

Fruit: serve with 1 cup fresh fruit

or

Pulse: double the lentil portion or add ½ cup chickpeas before refrigerating

Savory Mashed Chickpea Scramble—Quick!

Lean protein: **½ cup chickpeas, mashed**

Vegetable: **¼ cup each minced yellow onion, minced red bell pepper, and minced white button mushrooms; ½ cup baby spinach leaves; ¼ cup low-sodium organic vegetable broth**

Plant-based fat: **1 tablespoon extra-virgin olive oil**
Seasoning suggestion: **1 teaspoon minced garlic; 1 tablespoon fresh-squeezed lemon juice; ¹⁄₁₆ teaspoon each black pepper and cayenne pepper; 1 teaspoon salt-free Italian seasoning; 3 chopped fresh basil leaves**

In a medium sauté pan set over low heat, sauté the onion in the olive oil until it is translucent. Add the bell pepper, mushrooms, garlic, lemon juice, black pepper, cayenne, Italian seasoning, basil, and broth, and sauté the mixture until the pepper is tender. Stir in the chickpeas and spinach, and heat everything through, another 3 to 4 minutes.

Energy Accessory Ideas:
Whole grain: add ½ cup cooked red quinoa to sauté with the chickpeas
or
Starchy vegetable: serve with ½ cup oven-roasted, skin-on red or fingerling potatoes
or
Fruit: serve with 1 cup fresh fruit
or
Pulse: double the chickpea portion or add ½ cup lentils with the mashed chickpeas

Smoky Split Pea and Veggie Soup—*Make Ahead, Freeze & Reheat*

Lean protein: **½ cup cooked yellow split peas**
Vegetable: **¼ cup minced yellow onion, ½ cup low-sodium organic vegetable broth, ½ cup small cauliflower florets, ¼ cup minced celery, ½ cup baby spinach leaves**
Plant-based fat: **1 tablespoon extra-virgin coconut oil**
Seasoning suggestion: **1 teaspoon minced garlic, 1 teaspoon fresh-squeezed lemon juice, 1 teaspoon salt-free Italian seasoning, ¹⁄₁₆ teaspoon cumin, ¹⁄₁₆ teaspoon turmeric, ½ teaspoon smoked paprika**

In a medium saucepan set over low heat, sauté the onion in the coconut oil and 2 tablespoons of the broth until it is translucent. Stir in the remaining broth, cauliflower, garlic, lemon juice, Italian seasoning, cumin, tumeric, and paprika, and cook the mixture 3 to 4 minutes more. Stir in ½ cup of water and the celery and spinach. Raise the heat to high and bring the soup to a boil, then immediately reduce the heat and simmer it about 10 minutes. Add the split peas and heat them through; serve.

Energy Accessory Ideas:
Whole grain: add ½ cup cooked wild rice with the split peas
or

Starchy vegetable: add ½ cup oven-roasted, skin-on red potatoes with the split peas
or
Fruit: serve with 1 cup fresh fruit
or
Pulse: double the split pea portion or add ½ cup fava beans with the split peas

COOKING DRY SPLIT PEAS

It's easy to find canned options for nearly any bean as well as lentils and chickpeas. I've seen frozen black-eyed peas, lentils, and chickpeas, but I haven't been able to find canned or frozen split peas. While cooking split peas does require a little bit of time, it's fairly easy since they don't need hours of soaking. Here's how to do it.

- Step 1: Spread the split peas out on a clean dishtowel to inspect them. Pick out and throw away any debris, like pebbles or odd-looking peas.
- Step 2: Rinse the split peas in a colander under cold water.
- Step 3: In a medium saucepan set over high heat, boil 1½ cups of water for every 1 cup of split peas.
- Step 4: Add the split peas to the boiling water. Allow the water to return to a boil, then reduce it to a simmer, partially cover the saucepan, and cook the split peas until they are tender, 30 to 45 minutes (check after 30 minutes).
- Step 5: Drain them in a colander.
- Step 6: Use the cooked split peas or freeze ½ cup portions in BPA-free freezer baggies or containers (see page 270 for more about BPA). This allows you to thaw just what you need for your next recipe.

Garlic Basil White Bean Dip—*Quick!*, *Make Ahead,* *Take It with You*

....

Lean protein: **½ cup great northern beans**
Vegetable: **½ cup red bell pepper strips, ½ cup fresh whole radishes**
Plant-based fat: **1 tablespoon extra-virgin olive oil**
Seasoning suggestion: **1 teaspoon minced garlic, 1 tablespoon fresh-squeezed**
    lemon juice, ⅛ teaspoon black pepper, ½ tablespoon balsamic vinegar,
    ½ teaspoon salt-free Italian seasoning, 3 minced fresh basil leaves

In a blender or food processor, puree the beans with the oil, garlic, lemon juice, black pepper, and vinegar until the mixture is smooth, adding water 1 tablespoon at a time to thin if needed. Stir in the Italian seasoning and fresh basil. Serve the dip with the raw veggies.

Energy Accessory Ideas:

Whole grain: serve with 1 serving (according to the package) 100 percent whole-grain
    crackers
or
Starchy vegetable: serve with 1 cup baby carrots or carrot sticks
or
Fruit: serve with 1 cup fresh fruit
or
Pulse: serve with ½ cup Oven-Roasted Chickpeas (see page 175)

Garlic Rosemary Roasted Vegetables and Chickpeas

....

Lean protein: **½ cup cooked chickpeas**
Vegetable: **¼ cup each chopped red onion, chopped red bell pepper, chopped**
    eggplant, and small whole button mushrooms
Plant-based fat: **1 tablespoon extra-virgin olive oil**
Seasoning suggestion: **½ teaspoon minced garlic, 1 teaspoon fresh-squeezed**
    lemon juice, 1/16 teaspoon black pepper, 1 teaspoon minced fresh rosemary

Preheat the oven to 350°F. In a medium bowl, whisk together the olive oil, lemon juice, and black pepper. Place the chickpeas, onion, bell pepper, eggplant, and mushrooms on a baking sheet and rub or brush everything with the lemon-pepper oil. Bake the vegetables for 10 minutes, then sprinkle them with the rosemary and continue roasting them for 10 minutes.

Energy Accessory Ideas:

Whole grain: toss the roasted vegetables and chickpeas with ½ cup cooked brown
    rice penne
or

Starchy vegetable: serve with ½ cup oven-roasted fingerling potatoes or Baked
  Purple Sweet Potato [see page 174]
or
Fruit: serve with 1 cup fresh fruit
or
Pulse: double the chickpea portion

Mushroom and Cannellini Bean "Quiche"—Make Ahead, Take It with You, Freeze & Reheat

Lean protein: **½ cup cannellini beans**
Vegetable: **¾ cup minced white button mushrooms, ¼ cup minced white onion,
  ¼ cup low-sodium organic vegetable broth**
Plant-based fat: **1 tablespoon extra-virgin coconut oil**
Seasoning suggestion: **½ teaspoon minced garlic; ¹⁄₁₆ teaspoon each ground black
  and ground white pepper**

Preheat the oven to 350°F. In a medium sauté pan set over low heat, sauté the
mushrooms, onion, and garlic in the coconut oil until the onion is translucent. In
a blender, puree the beans with the broth and white and black pepper. Scrape
the bean mixture into a small [5-inch diameter] pie tin and fold in the mushroom
mixture. Bake the quiche for 25 minutes.

Energy Accessory Ideas:
Whole grain: add ½ cup quinoa to the mixture before baking
or
Starchy vegetable: serve with 1 cup cooked spaghetti squash or ½ cup Baked Purple
  Sweet Potato [see page 174]
or
Fruit: serve with 1 cup fresh fruit
or
Pulse: serve with ½ cup lima beans

Black-Eyed Pea Ginger Stir-Fry—Quick!, Make Ahead, Freeze & Reheat

Lean protein: **½ cup cooked black-eyed peas**
Vegetable: **¼ cup minced yellow onion, ¼ cup low-sodium organic vegetable
  broth, ¼ cup green bell pepper, ¼ cup red bell pepper, ¼ cup fresh whole
  snow peas**

Plant-based fat: **1 tablespoon extra-virgin coconut oil**

Seasoning suggestion: **1 teaspoon minced garlic, ¼ teaspoon grated fresh ginger, 1 tablespoon brown rice vinegar, ¼ teaspoon grated orange zest, ⅛ teaspoon black pepper**

In a medium sauté pan set over high heat, sauté the onion in the coconut oil and broth until it is translucent. Add the bell peppers, snow peas, garlic, ginger, vinegar, zest, and black pepper, and sauté the mixture until the bell peppers are slightly tender.

Energy Accessory Ideas:

Whole grain: serve over ½ cup cooked brown rice
or
Starchy vegetable: serve over 1 cup cooked spaghetti squash
or
Fruit: serve with 1 cup fresh fruit or add seedless orange slices to the stir-fry
or
Pulse: double the black-eyed pea portion

Cannellini Bean and Vegetable "Lasagna"—*Make Ahead, Freeze & Reheat*

Lean protein: **½ cup cooked cannellini beans**

Vegetable: **1 roma tomato, cut into thin rounds; 1 medium zucchini, sliced into ¼-inch rounds; 1 large whole portobello mushroom cap; 2 tablespoons minced red onion**

Plant-based fat: **1 tablespoon extra-virgin olive oil**

Seasoning suggestion: **1 teaspoon minced garlic, 3 or 4 chopped fresh basil leaves, ½ teaspoon salt-free Italian seasoning, ⅛ teaspoon black pepper, ¹⁄₁₆ teaspoon cayenne pepper**

Preheat the oven to 400°F. Place the tomato and zucchini slices and the mushroom on a baking sheet and brush or rub them with half of the olive oil. Roast them for 15 minutes. Meanwhile, in a blender or food processor, puree the beans with the remaining olive oil, garlic, and 1 tablespoon of water. Transfer the bean puree to a bowl and fold in the onion, basil, Italian seasoning, black pepper, and cayenne. Remove the vegetables from the oven, and on a second baking sheet, layer the vegetables with the beans: with the mushroom as the base, layer beans, then zucchini, then more beans, then tomatoes. Return the "lasagna" to the oven for 15 minutes.

Energy Accessory Ideas:

Whole grain: serve with ½ cup cooked 100 percent whole-grain penne
or

Starchy vegetable: serve with 1 cup cooked spaghetti squash
or
Fruit: serve with 1 cup fresh fruit
or
Pulse: serve with ½ cup Oven-Roasted Chickpeas (see page 175)

Black Bean Almond Ginger Satay—*Quick!, Make Ahead, Freeze & Reheat*

Lean protein: **½ cup black beans**
Vegetable: **¼ cup minced yellow onion, ¼ cup low-sodium organic vegetable broth, ¼ cup minced red bell pepper, ¼ cup shredded purple cabbage, ¼ cup minced white button mushrooms**
Plant-based fat: **2 tablespoons almond butter**
Seasoning suggestion: **½ teaspoon minced garlic, ½ teaspoon grated fresh ginger, ⅛ teaspoon ground turmeric, ⅛ teaspoon crushed red pepper flakes**

In a medium sauté pan set over low heat, sauté the onion in the broth until it is translucent. Add the garlic, bell pepper, cabbage, and mushrooms, and sauté the vegetables 2 to 3 more minutes. Add the ginger, turmeric, crushed red pepper, almond butter, and 2 tablespoons of water, and stir until everything is combined. Add the beans and heat them through; serve.

Energy Accessory Ideas:
Whole grain: serve over ½ cup cooked 100 percent whole-grain buckwheat soba noodles
or
Starchy vegetable: serve over ½ cup each shredded raw carrots and jicama
or
Fruit: serve with 1 cup fresh fruit
or
Pulse: double the black bean portion

Cayenne Pepper Cilantro Pinto Bean Dip—*Quick!, Make Ahead, Take It with You*

Lean protein: **½ cup pinto beans**
Vegetable: **¼ cup minced yellow onion; ¼ cup low-sodium organic vegetable broth; ½ cup each red bell pepper strips and chopped celery**
Plant-based fat: **¼ medium avocado, chopped**

Seasoning suggestion: ½ **teaspoon minced garlic,** ¹⁄₁₆ **teaspoon cumin,**
   ¹⁄₁₆ **teaspoon cayenne pepper, 1 teaspoon minced jalapeño, 1 teaspoon**
   chopped fresh cilantro

In a medium sauté pan set over low heat, sauté the onion in the broth until it is translucent. Stir in the beans, garlic, cumin, cayenne, jalapeño, and cilantro, and heat everything through, about 2 to 3 minutes. Transfer the bean mixture to a food processor and puree it with 2 tablespoons of water until it is smooth. Spoon the dip into a small dish, garnish it with the avocado, and serve it with the raw veggies.

Energy Accessory Ideas:

Whole grain: serve with ½ cup oven-roasted or heated frozen organic corn
or
Starchy vegetable: serve with 1 cup baby carrots or carrot sticks
or
Fruit: serve with 1 cup fresh fruit
or
Pulse: serve with ½ cup black beans on the side

Baked Chickpea Cakes over Sesame Arugula
....

Lean protein: ½ **cup chickpeas**
Vegetable: ¼ **cup chopped baby spinach leaves, 2 tablespoons minced yellow**
   onion, 1 cup arugula, ¼ cup halved grape tomatoes
Plant-based fat: **2 tablespoons tahini**
Seasoning suggestion: **2 teaspoons Dijon mustard, 2 teaspoons fresh-squeezed**
   lemon juice, 1 teaspoon minced garlic, ¹⁄₁₆ teaspoon cayenne pepper

Preheat the oven to 350°F. Mist a baking sheet with an olive oil–based nonstick spray. In a medium bowl, lightly mash the chickpeas and stir in the spinach, onion, mustard, 1 teaspoon of the lemon juice, garlic, and 1 teaspoon of water. Form the mixture into two round, flattened cakes, place them on the baking sheet, and bake them for 5 minutes on each side. Whisk the remaining lemon juice, cayenne, and 1 tablespoon of water into the tahini, and toss the dressing with the arugula. Place the arugula on a plate, top it with the tomatoes and chickpea cakes, and serve.

Energy Accessory Ideas:

Whole grain: sprinkle the arugula with ½ cup cooked quinoa or ¼ cup Toasted Quinoa
   [see page 174]
or
Starchy vegetable: serve with ½ cup Oven-Roasted Sweet Potato "Fries" [see page
   175] or Baked Purple Sweet Potato [see page 174]
or

Fruit: serve with 1 cup fresh fruit

or

Pulse: add ½ cup cooked lentils to the salad

Black Bean Avocado Cilantro Hummus—*Quick!*, Make Ahead, Take It with You

Lean protein: **½ cup black beans**
Vegetable: **½ cup small broccoli florets, ½ cup grape tomatoes**
Plant-based fat: **¼ medium avocado**
Seasoning suggestion: **½ teaspoon minced garlic, 1 tablespoon fresh-squeezed lime juice, 1/16 teaspoon cayenne pepper, 1 tablespoon minced fresh cilantro, 1/16 teaspoon cumin, 1 teaspoon minced jalapeño**

In a blender or food processor, puree the black beans with the avocado, garlic, lime juice, cayenne, cilantro, cumin, jalapeño, and 1 tablespoon of water until it is smooth. Serve the hummus with the raw veggies.

Energy Accessory Ideas:

Whole grain: serve with 1 serving (according to the package) 100 percent whole-grain crackers

or

Starchy vegetable: serve with 1 cup baby carrots or carrot sticks

or

Fruit: serve with 1 cup fresh fruit

or

Pulse: serve with ½ cup Oven-Roasted Chickpeas (see page 175)

White Bean and Kale Soup—*Make Ahead*, Freeze & Reheat

Lean protein: **½ cup great northern beans**
Vegetable: **¼ cup minced yellow onion; ½ cup low-sodium organic vegetable broth; 1 cup chopped kale; 1 roma tomato, diced**
Plant-based fat: **1 tablespoon extra-virgin olive oil**
Seasoning suggestion: **1 teaspoon minced garlic, 1 teaspoon fresh-squeezed lemon juice, ½ teaspoon salt-free Italian seasoning, ½ teaspoon smoked paprika, 1/8 teaspoon black pepper, 1 teaspoon balsamic vinegar**

In a medium saucepan set over low heat, sauté the onion in the olive oil and 2 tablespoons of the broth until it is translucent. Stir in the remaining broth, kale, garlic, lemon juice, Italian seasoning, paprika, pepper, and vinegar, and heat the mixture for 3 to 4 more minutes. Stir in ½ cup of water and the tomato, raise the heat and bring the soup to a boil, then immediately reduce the heat to medium-low and simmer the soup for about 10 minutes. Add the beans and heat them through; serve.

Energy Accessory Ideas:
Whole grain: add ½ cup cooked wild rice with the beans
or
Starchy vegetable: add ½ cup oven-roasted, skin-on red potatoes with the beans
or
Fruit: serve with 1 cup fresh fruit
or
Pulse: double the bean portion or add ½ cup lentils

Curried Lentil Lettuce Cups—*Quick!, Take It with You*
....

Lean protein: **½ cup lentils**
Vegetable: **¼ cup minced yellow onion; ¼ cup low-sodium organic vegetable broth; 1 small roma tomato, minced; 3 or 4 large outer leaves romaine lettuce**
Plant-based fat: **1 tablespoon extra-virgin coconut oil**
Seasoning suggestion: **2 teaspoons fresh-squeezed lemon juice; ½ teaspoon minced garlic; ¹⁄₁₆ teaspoon each ground coriander, cumin, turmeric, cinnamon, and black pepper**

In a medium sauté pan set over low heat, sauté the onion in the coconut oil and broth until it is translucent. Add the tomato, lemon juice, garlic, coriander, cumin, tumeric, cinnamon, and pepper, and stir 3 to 4 more minutes; add the lentils and heat them through. Fill the romaine leaves with the mixture and serve.

Energy Accessory Ideas:
Whole grain: add ½ cup cooked wild rice to sauté with the lentils
or
Starchy vegetable: serve with ½ cup cubed oven-baked, skin-on red potatoes, warm or chilled
or
Fruit: serve with 1 cup fresh fruit
or
Pulse: serve with ½ cup Oven-Roasted Chickpeas [see page 175]

Savory Lentil and Mushroom Stuffed Pepper— Make Ahead, Take It with You, Freeze & Reheat

Lean protein: **½ cup lentils**

Vegetable: **1 large whole red bell pepper, ¼ cup minced yellow onion, ¼ cup low-sodium organic vegetable broth, ½ cup minced white button mushrooms, ¼ cup finely chopped baby spinach leaves**

Plant-based fat: **1 tablespoon extra-virgin coconut oil**

Seasoning suggestion: **1 teaspoon minced garlic, ½ teaspoon salt-free Italian seasoning, ⅛ teaspoon crushed red pepper flakes, ¹⁄₁₆ teaspoon black pepper**

Preheat the oven to 375°F. Slice off the top of the bell pepper. Remove and discard the seeds and inner membranes, and set the pepper and its top aside. In a medium pan set over low heat, sauté the onion in the coconut oil and broth until it is translucent. Add the mushrooms, garlic, Italian seasoning, crushed red pepper, and black pepper, and sauté the mixture 2 or 3 more minutes. Add the lentils and spinach, and heat everything through. Spoon the mixture into the bell pepper and place it in a small baking dish; cover the dish with foil and bake it for 20 minutes. Remove the foil and bake the pepper 10 more minutes.

Energy Accessory Ideas:

Whole grain: add ½ cup cooked quinoa to the stuffing mixture

or

Starchy vegetable: serve with 1 cup cooked spaghetti squash

or

Fruit: serve with 1 cup fresh fruit

or

Pulse: serve with ½ cup Oven-Roasted Chickpeas (see page 175)

Pulse on the Go—Quick!, Make Ahead, Take It with You

Lean protein: **½ cup Oven-Roasted Chickpeas (see page 175)**

Vegetable: **½ cup each grape tomatoes and green or red bell pepper strips, or 1 cup On-the-Go Slaw (see page 175)**

Plant-based fat: **10 Mediterranean olives**

Pack all the ingredients in a sealable container and place the container in a stay-cold portable sack (if you pack the slaw, remember to bring a fork!).

Energy Accessory Ideas:

Whole grain: serve with 1 serving (according to the package) 100 percent whole-grain crackers or 3 cups Oil-Free Popped Popcorn (see page 175)

or

Starchy vegetable: add 1 cup carrot sticks

or

Fruit: serve with 1 cup fresh fruit

or

Pulse: double the chickpea portion or omit the olives and use hummus as a dip for the raw veggies

RESTAURANT OPTIONS

The seven meals that follow are just a sample of the types of options for eating out that fit the plan. In other words, it's by no means an exhaustive list. Restaurants change their menus regularly, and most are extremely accommodating to special requests, so as you identify new options or meals that fit from your favorite establishments, please share them with me at @CynthiaSass on Twitter or www.facebook.com/CynthiaSassFans.

Chipotle: Salad

Lean protein: **chicken or black beans or pinto beans**
Vegetable: **romaine lettuce, fajita vegetables, mild salsa**
Plant-based fat: **guacamole**

Order a salad made with romaine (no dressing), fajita vegetables, your lean protein choice, mild salsa, and guacamole. For the energy accessory, add either black beans, pinto beans, brown rice, or corn salsa, or pair the salad with your own serving of fresh fruit.

Panera Bread: Power Chicken Hummus Bowl

Lean protein: **chicken in the salad**
Vegetable: **spinach, cucumbers, tomatoes, onions in the salad**
Plant-based fat: **cilantro hummus**

Order the salad as is. This meal comes with hummus as the energy accessory.

California Pizza Kitchen: Roasted Veggie Salad

Lean protein: **grilled chicken breast or shrimp or salmon or black beans**
Vegetable: **romaine lettuce and roasted vegetables**
Plant-based fat: **avocado**

Order the salad with no dressing and your lean protein of choice, and ask for balsamic vinegar on the side. Don't worry: between the vinegar and avocado, you'll have plenty to coat and flavor the salad. This salad includes corn as an energy accessory.

PF Chang's: Shanghai Shrimp with Garlic Sauce

Lean protein: **shrimp in the dish**
Vegetable: **broccoli and snow peas in the dish**
Plant-based fat: **oil in the sauce**

Order this dish as is, with brown rice. Serve yourself ½ cup of brown rice, about the size of half a tennis ball, as the energy accessory.

Ruby Tuesday: Fit & Trim Grilled Salmon

Lean protein: **salmon**
Vegetable: **grilled zucchini in the dish**
Plant-based fat: **oil in the dish**

Order this meal as is. This dish comes with roasted spaghetti squash as the energy accessory.

Au Bon Pain: Vegetarian Deluxe Salad

Lean protein: **garbanzo beans in the salad**
Vegetable: **romaine lettuce, fire-roasted red and yellow bell peppers, tomatoes, cucumbers, carrots, and red onions in the salad**
Plant-based fat: **olives in the salad**

Order the salad without the feta cheese and dressing; ask for balsamic vinegar on the side. Ask for extra garbanzo beans for your energy accessory.

The Cheesecake Factory: SkinnyLicious® Grilled Chicken Tostado Salad

Lean protein: **grilled chicken in the salad**
Vegetable: **mixed greens and onions in the salad, salsa as garnish**
Plant-based fat: **avocado in the salad**

Order the salad without the dressing, sour cream, or avocado cream. Ask for avocado in place of the avocado cream. The meal comes with either black beans or corn for the energy accessory; choose only one and ask that the other be left off.

FREQUENTLY USED WARDROBE PIECES

I've referred to the following recipes throughout this chapter. Here you can see just how simple they are. They really just add a few more steps to your meal preparation.

Baked Purple Sweet Potato

Preheat the oven to 350°F. Wash 1 purple sweet potato and pat it dry. Wrap it in aluminum foil and bake it for 90 minutes. Unwrap the potato, scoop out its flesh, and use it or refrigerate it and enjoy it chilled.

Toasted Quinoa

Preheat the oven to 350°F. Rinse ¼ cup uncooked quinoa in a fine-mesh sieve under running water for about a minute. Pat the quinoa dry, then lightly mist it with an olive oil–based nonstick spray (or your own mister filled with extra-virgin olive oil). Spread the oiled quinoa out on a baking sheet and toast it for 10 minutes.

Oven-Roasted Sweet Potato "Fries"

Preheat the oven to 450°F. Peel 1 small sweet potato and cut it into long, thin slices. Lightly mist the slices with an olive oil–based nonstick spray (or your own mister filled with extra-virgin olive oil). Spread the slices out on a baking sheet. Bake them for 15 minutes, then flip them with a spatula and bake them for 10 to 15 more minutes, until they are crisp.

Oil-Free Popped Popcorn

Place ¼ cup organic popcorn kernels in a brown paper bag. Close the bag and fold the top over a few times, then place the bag in a microwave and cook the kernels on high for 2½ minutes. Monitor the popcorn carefully, and remove it sooner if you hear the kernels stop popping.

Oven-Roasted Chickpeas

Preheat the oven to 350°F. Rinse and then lightly mist ½ cup canned chickpeas with an olive oil–based nonstick spray (or your own mister filled with extra-virgin olive oil). Spread the chickpeas out on a baking sheet and roast them for 10 minutes.

On-the-Go Slaw

In a sealable container, whisk together 1 tablespoon brown rice vinegar, 1 tablespoon 100 percent orange juice, ¼ teaspoon grated fresh ginger, ¼ teaspoon minced garlic, and 1/16 teaspoon black pepper. Add 1 cup shredded cabbage, zucchini, or broccoli, or a mixture. Seal the container, gently shake the mixture to coat everything, and refrigerate the slaw for at least 30 minutes.

Weekly Meal Plans and Shopping Lists

Though you're free to choose any of the meals in this chapter, I know some people prefer the convenience of following a preselected plan with an accompanying grocery list. I've put together four versions:

- A plan for omnivores (includes all animal-based proteins)
- A plan for vegans (without animal-derived ingredients)
- A plan for lacto-ovo vegetarians (includes eggs and dairy but no poultry or seafood)
- An omnivore plan that includes eggs but is gluten free and dairy free

Again, these are optional. They're simply sample plans you can use if you find them helpful.

If you want to streamline your meal planning and minimize your grocery trips, choose a couple of recipe favorites and repeat them for meals 1 and 2 for the whole week. For variety, mix things up for your third meal of the day. For example, for meal 1 you could alternate between the Mexi Omelet and the Strawberry Peanut Butter Smoothie. For meal 2, you could switch between Cheesy Cauliflower Casserole and California Chicken Salad.

Even repeating a single recipe all week for meal 1 is perfectly fine if you find this routine helpful. You can take the same approach for lunch. If your staple is a salad or a dish you can make ahead, like hummus, it's A-OK to choose one or two and enjoy them all week.

For meal 3, even if you don't prepare seven different recipes in a week, try to incorporate some variety. Just remember that one of your daily meals must include a serving of pulse, either a plus-pulse meal, with pulse as the energy accessory, or a pulse-as-protein option, in which pulse is the lean protein, such as Black Bean "Tacos" or Moroccan Lentil Soup. If you're short on time to prepare meal 3, scan the recipes for those marked *Quick!* Or if you have more time on the weekends, look for recipes designated *Make Ahead* or *Freeze & Reheat*.

I want you to feel great every day during this 30-day challenge, so if cooking and enjoying a variety of meals make you happy, by all means use the sample plans and grocery lists I've created. And if these plans and lists look too overwhelming or time-consuming, opt to keep it simple.

If a pared-down weekly meal plan works best for you, it may be easiest to bring this book with you to the market, with the pages marked for the recipes you want to make. Or photocopy the pages and take them with you. And please remember that you aren't limited to the recipes in this chapter. You can also use the do-it-yourself meal building strategy and lists in chapter 3 to craft your own meal selections using your favorite or staple foods.

7-Day Omnivore Plan [includes all animal-based proteins]

Day 1

Meal 1

California Omelet (page 113) with oven-roasted red potatoes as the energy accessory

Meal 2

Moroccan Lentil Soup (page 158) with a sliced fresh pear as the energy accessory (daily pulse)

Meal 3

Broccoli Cashew Chicken Stir-Fry (page 138) with brown rice as the energy accessory

Day 2

Meal 1

Almond Oatmeal (page 123) with oats as the energy accessory (daily pulse)

Meal 2

Pesto Egg Salad (page 114) with whole-grain crackers as the energy accessory

Meal 3

Garlicky Shrimp Scampi (page 150) with spaghetti squash as the energy accessory

Day 3

Meal 1

Strawberry Peanut Butter Smoothie (page 124) with strawberries as the energy accessory

Meal 2

Chilled Chicken Dijon Salad (page 140) with one slice of toasted 100 percent whole-grain bread as the energy accessory

Meal 3

Black Bean "Tacos" (page 158) with corn as the energy accessory (daily pulse)

Day 4

Meal 1

Savory Veggie Quiche (page 121) with green grapes as the energy accessory

Meal 2

Lemon Pepper Hummus (page 160) with baby carrots as the energy accessory (daily pulse)

Meal 3

Gingery Chicken and Veggie Almond Satay (page 143) with 100 percent whole-grain buckwheat soba noodles as the energy accessory

Day 5

Meal 1

Chocolate Raspberry Parfait (page 135) with raspberries as the energy accessory

Meal 2

Spinach Walnut Salad (page 120) with lentils as the energy accessory (daily pulse)

Meal 3

Salmon with Garlic Rosemary Roasted Vegetables (page 150) with wild rice as the energy accessory

Day 6

Meal 1

Lemon Mint Avocado Smoothie (page 132) with pineapple in the smoothie as the energy accessory

Meal 2

Baked Chickpea Cakes over Sesame Arugula (page 168) with quinoa as the energy accessory (daily pulse)

Meal 3

Cheesy Cauliflower Casserole (page 130) with green grapes as the energy accessory

Day 7

Meal 1

Savory Mashed Chickpea Scramble (page 161) with a sliced fresh apple as the energy accessory (daily pulse)

Meal 2

Basil Balsamic Tuna Salad (page 151) with Oven-Roasted Sweet Potato "Fries" (page 175) as the energy accessory

Meal 3

Simple Chicken Cacciatore (page 138) with whole-grain penne as the energy accessory

7-Day Omnivore Plan Grocery List

Fresh Produce

Vegetables

1 small vine-ripened tomato

2 roma tomatoes

1 large container grape tomatoes (2 cups needed)

4 large yellow onions

2 large red onions

1 large bunch or container spinach leaves (6 cups needed)

1 head or container romaine lettuce (6 or 7 large outer leaves needed)

1 bunch or container arugula (1 cup needed)

1 small bunch kale—buy loose or bagged if you can (only ½ cup chopped needed)

Purple cabbage—buy loose or bagged if you can (only ¼ cup shredded needed)

Cauliflower—buy loose or bagged if you can (only ½ cup florets needed)

1 head broccoli (2 cups florets needed)

1 small package (or loose) white button mushrooms (1 cup needed)

1 large zucchini

2 or 3 large red bell peppers

1 small green bell pepper

1 small yellow bell pepper

1 small jalapeño

1 cup whole snow peas

1 small spaghetti squash

2 medium red potatoes

1 small sweet potato

1 bag baby carrots

Fruit

1 pear, any type

1 apple, any type

1 bunch green grapes (2 cups needed)

1 cup raspberries (frozen is okay)

1 bag lemons (3 to 6)

1 organic lemon for zesting (dried organic lemon zest is okay as an alternative)

1 lime

Other

1 2-inch piece fresh ginger

1 small bunch flat-leaf parsley

1 small bunch cilantro

1 small bunch rosemary

1 small bunch mint

1 small bunch basil

2 avocados

Meat

1 pound cooked boneless skinless chicken breast

Seafood

4 ounces fresh wild salmon (frozen is okay as an alternative)

Refrigerated Items

2 dozen organic eggs, or 1 dozen organic eggs and 1 container organic liquid egg whites (if you prefer liquid whites for the recipes that do not call for hard-boiled eggs)

3 single-serving containers nonfat vanilla-flavored organic Greek yogurt

1 small container organic nonfat cottage cheese

Frozen Foods

1 small bag peeled deveined cooked medium shrimp

1 small bag strawberries

1 small bag pineapple

1 small bag organic corn

Canned Goods

1 15.5-ounce can lentils

1 15.5-ounce can black beans

1 15.5-ounce can chickpeas

1 3- or 5-ounce can chunk light tuna, packed in water (3 ounces needed)

Packaged/Shelf-Stable Products

1 32-ounce container low-sodium organic vegetable broth

1 jar extra-virgin coconut oil

1 small bottle extra-virgin olive oil

1 small bag unsalted cashews

1 small bag unsalted almonds

1 jar natural peanut butter

1 jar almond butter

1 jar tahini

1 box brown rice

1 box wild rice

1 box quinoa

1 small canister old-fashioned rolled oats

1 package 100 percent whole-grain buckwheat soba noodles

1 box 100 percent whole-grain penne

1 small loaf 100 percent whole-grain bread (only 1 slice needed)

1 package 100 percent whole-grain crackers

1 canister unsweetened pea protein powder

1 can olive oil–based cooking spray

1 small jar 100 percent vegetable juice (unless juicing your own from
fresh produce)

1 1-ounce bar dark chocolate (at least 70 percent cacao)

Dried/Jarred Seasonings

1 container ground black pepper

1 container cayenne pepper

1 container salt-free Italian seasoning

1 container ground cinnamon

1 container ground cumin

1 container ground turmeric

1 container ground coriander

1 container ground celery seed

1 container crushed red pepper flakes

1 4.25-ounce jar minced garlic in water

1 jar basil pesto

1 jar Dijon mustard

1 bottle balsamic vinegar

7-Day Vegan Plan [no animal-derived ingredients]

Note: Every meal is a pulse meal, so I haven't designated the daily pulse.

Day 1

Meal 1

Savory Mashed Chickpea Scramble (page 161) with a sliced fresh apple as the energy accessory

Meal 2

Moroccan Lentil Soup (page 158) with wild rice as the energy accessory

Meal 3

Cannellini Bean and Vegetable "Lasagna" (page 166) with spaghetti squash as the energy accessory

Day 2

Meal 1

Cherry Chocolate Green Goddess Smoothie (page 160) with cherries as the energy accessory

Meal 2

Black Bean "Tacos" (page 158) with corn as the energy accessory

Meal 3

Black-Eyed Pea Ginger Stir-Fry (page 165) with brown rice as the energy accessory

Day 3

Meal 1

Almond Oatmeal (page 123) with oats as the energy accessory

Meal 2

Lemon Pepper Hummus (page 160) with baby carrots as the energy accessory

Meal 3

White Bean and Kale Soup (page 169) with red grapes as the energy accessory

Day 4

Meal 1

Mushroom and Cannellini Bean "Quiche" (page 165) with a sliced fresh pear as the energy accessory

Meal 2

Chilled Basil Balsamic Lentil Salad (page 161) with quinoa as the energy accessory

Meal 3

Garlic Rosemary Roasted Vegetables and Chickpeas (page 164) with red or fingerling potatoes as the energy accessory

Day 5

Meal 1

Mexi Omelet (page 118) with ½ cup mashed black beans in place of the egg and corn as the energy accessory

Meal 2

Garlic Basil White Bean Dip (page 164) with whole-grain crackers as the energy accessory

Meal 3

Smoky Split Pea and Veggie Soup (page 162) with wild rice as the energy accessory

Day 6

Meal 1

Green Goddess Smoothie (page 159) with mango as the energy accessory

Meal 2

Curried Lentil Lettuce Cups (page 170) with Oil-Free Popped Popcorn (page 175) as the energy accessory

Meal 3

Black Bean Almond Ginger Satay (page 167) with 100 percent whole-grain buckwheat soba noodles as the energy accessory

Day 7

Meal 1

Cayenne Pepper Cilantro Pinto Bean Dip (page 167) with a sliced fresh apple as the energy accessory

Meal 2

Baked Chickpea Cakes over Sesame Arugula (page 168) with Oven-Roasted Sweet Potato "Fries" (page 175) as the energy accessory

Meal 3

Savory Lentil and Mushroom Stuffed Pepper (page 171) with quinoa as the energy accessory

7-Day Vegan Plan Grocery List

Fresh Produce

Vegetables

4 roma tomatoes

1 large container grape tomatoes (about 2 cups needed)

4 large yellow onions

2 large red onions

1 large white onion

1 small head celery

1 large bunch or container spinach leaves (4 cups needed)

1 head or container romaine lettuce (6 to 8 large outer leaves needed)

1 bunch or container arugula (1 cup needed)

1 small bunch kale—buy loose or bagged if you can (only 1 cup chopped needed)

Purple cabbage—buy loose or bagged if you can (only ¼ cup shredded needed)

Cauliflower—buy loose or bagged if you can (only 1 cup florets needed)

Broccoli—buy loose or bagged if you can (½ cup florets needed)

1 small package (or loose) white button mushrooms (about 2½ cups needed)

1 large whole portobello mushroom

1 medium zucchini

1 small eggplant

4 large red bell peppers

1 large green bell pepper

1 small cucumber

1 small bunch radishes (½ cup needed)

3 small jalapeños

¼ cup whole snow peas

1 small spaghetti squash

1 small bag red or fingerling potatoes—buy loose if you can (½ cup needed)

1 small sweet potato

1 bag baby carrots

Fruit

1 pear, any type

2 apples, any type

1 bunch red grapes (1 cup needed)

1 bag lemons (3 to 6)

1 organic lemon for zesting (dried organic lemon zest is okay as an alternative)

1 organic orange for zesting (dried organic orange zest is okay as an alternative)

2 limes

Other

1 4-inch piece fresh ginger

1 small bunch cilantro

1 small bunch rosemary

1 small bunch basil

4 avocados

Frozen Foods

1 small bag frozen cherries

1 small bag organic corn

1 bag frozen mango

Canned Goods

2 15.5-ounce cans lentils

1 15.5-ounce can cannellini beans

2 15.5-ounce cans black beans

1 15.5-ounce can pinto beans

2 15.5-ounce cans chickpeas

1 15.5-ounce can black-eyed peas

1 15.5-ounce can great northern beans

Packaged/Shelf-Stable Products

1 32-ounce container low-sodium organic vegetable broth

1 jar extra-virgin coconut oil

1 small bottle extra-virgin olive oil

1 small bag unsalted almonds

1 jar almond butter

1 jar tahini

1 box brown rice

1 box wild rice

1 box quinoa

1 small bag yellow split peas

1 small bag organic popcorn kernels

1 small canister old-fashioned rolled oats

1 package 100 percent whole-grain buckwheat soba noodles

1 package 100 percent whole-grain vegan crackers

1 canister unsweetened pea protein powder

1 can olive oil–based cooking spray

1 small jar 100 percent vegetable juice (unless juicing your own from fresh produce)

1 1-ounce bar dark chocolate (at least 70 percent cacao)

Dried/Jarred Seasonings

1 container ground black pepper

1 container ground white pepper

1 container cayenne pepper

1 container salt-free Italian seasoning

1 container ground cinnamon

1 container ground cumin

1 container ground turmeric

1 container ground coriander

1 container bay leaf

1 container paprika

1 container smoked paprika

1 container crushed red pepper flakes

1 4.25-ounce jar minced garlic in water

1 jar Dijon mustard

1 bottle balsamic vinegar

1 bottle brown rice vinegar

7-Day Lacto-Ovo Vegetarian Plan [includes eggs and dairy but no poultry or seafood]

Day 1

Meal 1

Mexi Omelet (page 118) with corn as the energy accessory

Meal 2

Lemon Pepper Hummus (page 160) with baby carrots as the energy accessory (daily pulse)

Meal 3

Cheesy Cauliflower Casserole (page 130) with wild rice as the energy accessory

Day 2

Meal 1

Pineapple Ginger Coconut Parfait (page 137) with pineapple as the energy accessory

Meal 2

Pesto Egg Salad (page 114) with whole-grain crackers as the energy accessory

Meal 3

Smoky Split Pea and Veggie Soup (page 162) with wild rice as the energy accessory (daily pulse)

Day 3

Meal 1

Blueberry Coconut Smoothie (page 126) with blueberries as the energy accessory

Meal 2

Black Bean "Tacos" (page 158) with corn as the energy accessory (daily pulse)

Meal 3

Roasted Vegetable "Lasagna" (page 132) with quinoa as the energy accessory

Day 4

Meal 1

Mushroom and Cannellini Bean "Quiche" (page 165) with a sliced fresh pear as the energy accessory (daily pulse)

Meal 2

Wilted Lemon Pepper Arugula Salad (page 114) with wild rice as the energy accessory

Meal 3

Cheesy Savory Stuffed Pepper (page 134) with spaghetti squash as the energy accessory

Day 5

Meal 1

Chocolate Raspberry Parfait (page 135) with raspberries as the energy accessory

Meal 2

Moroccan Lentil Soup (page 158) with wild rice as the energy accessory (daily pulse)

Meal 3

Gingery Egg Satay (page 115) with 100 percent whole-grain buckwheat soba noodles as the energy accessory

Day 6

Meal 1

Lemon Mint Avocado Smoothie (page 132) with pineapple in the smoothie as the energy accessory

Meal 2

Chilled Pesto Cheesy Salad (page 127) with quinoa as the energy accessory

Meal 3

Baked Chickpea Cakes over Sesame Arugula (page 168) with Oven-Roasted Sweet Potato "Fries" (page 175) as the energy accessory (daily pulse)

Day 7

Meal 1

Savory Veggie Quiche (page 121) with grapes as the energy accessory

Meal 2

Sesame Ricotta Dip (page 133) with whole-grain crackers as the energy accessory

Meal 3

White Bean and Kale Soup (page 169) with wild rice as the energy accessory (daily pulse)

7-Day Lacto-Ovo Vegetarian Plan Grocery List

Fresh Produce

Vegetables

  3 roma tomatoes

  1 large container grape tomatoes (2 cups needed)

  3 large yellow onions

  1 large red onion

  1 large white onion

  1 small head celery—buy loose or bagged if you can (only a few stalks needed)

  1 large bunch or container spinach leaves (about 4¼ cups needed)

  1 head or container romaine lettuce (6 or 7 large outer leaves needed)

  1 bunch or container arugula (3½ cups needed)

  1 small bunch kale—buy loose or bagged if you can (only 1½ cups chopped needed)

  Cabbage—buy loose or bagged if you can (only ¼ cup shredded needed)

  1 head cauliflower (1¾ cups florets needed)

  1 head broccoli (¼ cup florets needed)

  1 small package (or loose) white button mushrooms (about 1½ cups needed)

  1 large portobello mushroom

  2 medium zucchini

  3 large red bell peppers

  3 large green bell peppers

  2 small jalapeños

  ½ cup whole snow peas

  1 small spaghetti squash

  1 small sweet potato

  1 bag baby carrots

Fruit

 1 pear, any type

 1 bunch grapes, any type

 1 cup raspberries (frozen is okay as an alternative)

 1 bag lemons (3 to 6)

 1 organic lemon for zesting (dried organic lemon zest is okay as an
 alternative)

 1 lime

Other

 1 3-inch piece fresh ginger

 1 small bunch cilantro

 1 small bunch mint

 2 avocados

Refrigerated Items

 2 dozen organic eggs, or 1 dozen organic eggs and 1 container organic
 liquid egg whites (if you prefer liquid whites for the recipes that do
 not call for hard-boiled eggs)

 4 single-serving containers nonfat vanilla-flavored organic Greek
 yogurt

 1 16-ounce container organic nonfat cottage cheese

 1 small container organic nonfat ricotta cheese

Frozen Foods

 1 small bag blueberries

 1 small bag pineapple

 1 small bag organic corn

Canned Goods

 1 15.5-ounce can lentils

 1 15.5-ounce can black beans

 1 15.5-ounce can chickpeas

 1 15.5-ounce can cannellini beans

 1 15.5-ounce can great northern beans

Packaged/Shelf-Stable Products

1 32-ounce container low-sodium organic vegetable broth

1 jar extra-virgin coconut oil

1 small bottle extra-virgin olive oil

1 jar natural peanut butter

1 jar tahini

1 box wild rice

1 box quinoa

1 small bag yellow split peas

1 package 100 percent whole-grain buckwheat soba noodles

1 package 100 percent whole-grain crackers

1 small jar 100 percent vegetable juice (unless juicing your own from fresh produce)

1 small bag unsweetened shredded or flaked coconut

1 1-ounce bar dark chocolate (at least 70 percent cacao)

Dried/Jarred Seasonings

1 container ground black pepper

1 container ground white pepper

1 container cayenne pepper

1 container salt-free Italian seasoning

1 container ground cinnamon

1 container ground cumin

1 container ground turmeric

1 container ground coriander

1 container bay leaf

1 container paprika

1 container smoked paprika

1 container crushed red pepper flakes

1 4.25-ounce jar minced garlic in water

1 jar basil pesto

1 jar Dijon mustard

1 bottle balsamic vinegar

7-Day Omnivore Gluten-Free and Dairy-Free Plan

(includes eggs)

Day 1

Meal 1

California Omelet (page 113) with oven-roasted red potatoes as the energy accessory

Meal 2

Moroccan Lentil Soup (page 158) with a sliced fresh pear as the energy accessory (daily pulse)

Meal 3

Broccoli Cashew Chicken Stir-Fry (page 138) with brown rice as the energy accessory

Day 2

Meal 1

Almond Oatmeal (page 123) with oats as the energy accessory (daily pulse)

Meal 2

Southwest Egg Salad (page 121) with organic corn as the energy accessory

Meal 3

Garlicky Shrimp Scampi (page 150) with spaghetti squash as the energy accessory

Day 3

Meal 1

Green Goddess Smoothie (page 159) with mango as the energy accessory

Meal 2

Chilled Chicken Dijon Salad (page 140) with wild rice as the energy accessory

Meal 3

Black Bean "Tacos" (page 158) with corn as the energy accessory (daily pulse)

Day 4

Meal 1

Savory Veggie Quiche (page 121) with green grapes as the energy accessory

Meal 2

Lemon Pepper Hummus (page 160) with baby carrots as the energy accessory (daily pulse)

Meal 3

Gingery Chicken and Veggie Almond Satay (page 143) with 100 percent whole-grain buckwheat soba noodles as the energy accessory

Day 5

Meal 1

Ginger Broccoli Scramble (page 118) with a fresh orange as the energy accessory

Meal 2

Spinach Walnut Salad (page 120) with lentils as the energy accessory (daily pulse)

Meal 3

Salmon with Garlic Rosemary Roasted Vegetables (page 150) with wild rice as the energy accessory

Day 6

Meal 1

Cherry Chocolate Green Goddess Smoothie (page 160) with cherries as the energy accessory

Meal 2

Baked Chickpea Cakes over Sesame Arugula (page 168) with quinoa as the energy accessory (daily pulse)

Meal 3

Simple Tom Yum Shrimp Soup (page 153) with a sliced fresh pear as the energy accessory

Day 7

Meal 1

Savory Mashed Chickpea Scramble (page 161) with a sliced fresh apple
as the energy accessory (daily pulse)

Meal 2

Basil Balsamic Tuna Salad (page 151) with Oven-Roasted Sweet Potato
"Fries" (page 175) as the energy accessory

Meal 3

Simple Chicken Cacciatore (page 138) with spaghetti squash as the
energy accessory

7-Day Omnivore Gluten-Free and Dairy-Free Plan
(includes eggs) **Grocery List**

*Note: Check each packaged food to ensure that it is gluten free and not made
in a facility that also processes wheat or other gluten-containing foods.*

Fresh Produce

Vegetables

1 small vine-ripened tomato

2 roma tomatoes

1 large container grape tomatoes (about 2½ cups needed)

4 large yellow onions

2 large red onions

1 large white onion

1 large bunch or container spinach leaves (about 6 cups needed)

1 head or container romaine lettuce (6 or 7 large outer leaves needed)

1 bunch or container arugula (1 cup needed)

1 small bunch kale—buy loose or bagged if you can (only ½ cup
chopped needed)

Purple cabbage—buy loose or bagged if you can (only ¼ cup shredded
needed)

Cauliflower—buy loose or bagged if you can (only ½ cup florets
needed)

1 head broccoli (about 3 cups florets needed)

1 small package (or loose) white button mushrooms (about 2 cups needed)

1 medium zucchini

2 large red bell peppers

2 large green bell peppers

1 small yellow bell pepper

2 small jalapeños

1 cup whole snow peas

2 small spaghetti squash

2 medium red-skinned potatoes

1 small sweet potato

1 bag baby carrots

Fruit

2 pears, any type

1 apple, any type

1 orange, any type

1 bunch green grapes (1 cup needed)

1 bag lemons (3 to 6)

1 organic lemon for zesting (dried organic lemon zest is okay as an alternative)

3 limes

Other

1 4-inch piece fresh ginger

1 small bunch flat-leaf parsley

1 small bunch cilantro

1 small bunch rosemary

1 small bunch basil

3 avocados

Meat

1 pound cooked boneless skinless chicken breast

Seafood

4 ounces fresh wild salmon (frozen is okay as an alternative)

Refrigerated Items

2 dozen organic eggs, or 1 dozen organic eggs and 1 container organic liquid egg whites (if you prefer liquid whites for the recipes that do not call for hard-boiled eggs)

Frozen Foods

1 small bag peeled deveined cooked medium shrimp

1 small bag cherries

1 small bag mango

1 small bag organic corn

Canned Goods

1 15.5-ounce can lentils

1 15.5-ounce can black beans

1 15.5-ounce can chickpeas

1 3- or 5-ounce can chunk light tuna, packed in water (3 ounces needed)

Packaged/Shelf-Stable Products

1 32-ounce container low-sodium organic vegetable broth

1 jar extra-virgin coconut oil

1 small bottle extra-virgin olive oil

1 small bag unsalted cashews

1 small bag unsalted walnuts

1 small bag unsalted almonds

1 jar almond butter

1 jar tahini

1 box brown rice

1 box wild rice

1 box quinoa

1 small canister old-fashioned gluten-free rolled oats

1 package 100 percent whole-grain buckwheat soba noodles

1 canister unsweetened pea protein powder

1 olive oil–based cooking spray

1 small jar 100 percent vegetable juice (unless juicing your own from fresh produce)

1 1-ounce bar dark chocolate (at least 70 percent cacao)

Dried/Jarred Seasonings

1 container ground black pepper

1 container cayenne pepper

1 container salt-free Italian seasoning

1 container ground cinnamon

1 container ground cumin

1 container ground turmeric

1 container ground coriander

1 container ground celery seed

1 container kaffir lime leaf

1 container lemongrass

1 container crushed red pepper flakes

1 4.25-ounce jar minced garlic in water

1 jar Dijon mustard

1 bottle balsamic vinegar

HOW TO SHOP TO REDUCE YOUR EXPOSURE TO HARMFUL CHEMICALS—AND SAVE MONEY TO BOOT!

As you can see, my plan is primarily based on fresh foods. These foods are not only unprocessed and nutrient rich, but many of them also are unpackaged. Buying fewer packaged products is another important way to protect your health. According to a recent study published in the *British Medical Journal,* the synthetic chemicals used in food processing and packaging can leach into food. That means eating more foods that come from a box, can, bag, or container of some kind can lead to ingesting low levels of these substances over a lifetime. Some chemicals, such as bisphenol A (BPA), have been shown to disrupt hormone production and balance. Others, like formaldehyde, are linked to increased cancer risk. I know it's not practical to eliminate packaged foods completely, but in addition to purchasing more fresh produce, you can cut back in other ways. For example

- Shop the bulk section. You can buy many of the healthy staples you'll need for this plan in bulk, including oats, brown and wild rice, quinoa, popcorn, nuts, seeds, dried herbs, and pulses. Bulk buying saves you money, because the cost of packaging is passed on to consumers. It's also a great way to avoid waste, because you can bring home only what you need. Storing these foods in sealed glass containers reduces the number of products that sit in your cupboards wrapped in packaging. If you ever forget prep instructions because the packaging is missing, like how much water to add to wild rice, just hop online to find out.

- Grow or buy potted herbs. Fresh herbs can be some of the most expensive items on your grocery list, but there are more affordable options. The first is to grow your own, using kits you can buy online or at stores that sell gardening products. Or buy small pots of living herbs, like basil, mint, rosemary, cilantro, and parsley. Most grocery stores now sell them in the produce section, and I almost always find them at my local farmers' market. You can't get much fresher than herbs still rooted in soil, and small plants can cost as little as $2. Keep them alive, snip off just what you need for a recipe, and your investment can last a good while.

- Make it yourself. Whipping up some foods you may typically buy in packages, such as whole-grain bread, crackers, or nonfat Greek yogurt, can be fun projects to take on with kids, friends, or family members. The Internet is chock full of free recipes, including versions that are gluten free or vegan. If you're up for an adventure, give it a go!

[6]

Desserts

Let's face it: few of us can go through life without enjoying a treat now and then, right? Well, I'm happy to tell you that in addition to the meals that include chocolate in chapter 5, like the Chocolate Raspberry Parfait (page 135), you can build *additional* splurges into your eating plan and continue to shed pounds (and keep them off). But if you're going to indulge, why not satisfy your sweet tooth while also reaping health and nutritional benefits?

In this chapter I present recipes for four outrageously delicious sweet treats: intense, dark-chocolate brownie bites; fudgy, melt-in-your-mouth chocolate truffles; creamy cherry coconut pops; and my favorite, earthy, aromatic spiced pumpkin mini muffins. Each is stealthily made with the superstar of my plan: pulses! Don't worry. You won't detect the flavor of the pureed beans or garbanzo bean (chickpea) flour, which seamlessly blend in with the recipes' other ingredients. But you will benefit from the nutrients, fiber, and antioxidants these pulses pack, as well as the satiety boost they provide, so you'll feel satisfied with a reasonable portion. And you can use any of the pudding recipes from the Rapid Pulse as desserts too (the dark chocolate version was a favorite with the women who tested this plan—and their kids!). Treats made with refined flour and excess sugar can trigger lingering hunger, sluggishness, and a stoked-up sweet tooth, but these delights will leave you feeling full, satisfied, light, and energized.

How often can you indulge? After you complete the four-day Rapid Pulse, you can include sweet treats in up to two meals a week on nonconsecutive days. You have the option of choosing either three mini muffins,

THE MINI TRICK

When I created these recipes, my first instinct was to have you bake a pan of brownies and loaf of pumpkin bread, and slice them up. Instead, I've tailored the recipes for smaller, individual portions, including mini muffins and brownies. So, instead of eating one large piece of pumpkin bread, you eat three mini pumpkin muffins. I've gone this route because of an intriguing Arizona State University study, which found that eating smaller pieces boosts satiety more than eating one larger piece of the exact same amount of food. This may be because smaller tidbits, with spaces in between, visually look like more food than one larger portion. It may also be that bringing your hand to your mouth more times tricks your brain into thinking you've eaten more. In either case, this approach works! If you don't already have a mini muffin pan, which is roughly 9 by 15 inches and holds twenty-four muffins, I hope you'll see buying one as a worthy investment.

two truffles, or one pop or pudding as your energy accessory or second energy accessory, based on the results of your My Energy Needs quiz on page 87.

Many of my clients choose specific days of the week to build in splurges so they know they have something to look forward to. Some select "hump day" (Wednesday), because it breaks up the week, and Saturday, which feels like a mini vacation day, perfect for enjoying a special treat. For others, a once-a-week ritual feels like a better fit, so they might choose to indulge every Friday night or Sunday afternoon. If a week goes by and you don't feel a hankering for a treat, that's A-OK as well. The purpose of my treat recipes is simply to offer you healthier ways to satisfy your sweet tooth and take advantage once again of the power of pulses.

Pulse Brownie Bites

½ cup garbanzo bean (chickpea) flour
½ cup almond flour
½ cup organic cane sugar
½ cup unsweetened cocoa powder
½ teaspoon baking powder
½ teaspoon salt
½ cup water
½ cup extra-virgin olive oil
1 teaspoon pure vanilla extract
½ cup banana slices
¼ cup chopped dark chocolate

Preheat the oven to 350°F. In a large bowl, stir together the garbanzo bean flour, almond flour, sugar, cocoa powder, baking powder, and salt. In a blender, combine the water, olive oil, vanilla, and banana; blend the mixture until it is smooth. Fold the wet ingredients into the dry mix to form a smooth, uniform batter. Stir in the chocolate. Spoon 1 tablespoon of batter into each of 24 paper cup–lined mini muffin cups. Bake for 15 minutes, until a toothpick inserted into a brownie comes out clean. Let the brownie bites cool for at least 10 minutes. (Note: wrapped up, these will keep for three days at room temperature. They also freeze well. Just defrost them at room temperature for about 25 minutes before enjoying.)

Makes 24 brownie bites, or 8 servings

Vanilla Cinnamon Pulse Truffles

¼ cup chopped dark chocolate
¼ cup very hot water (almost boiling)
½ tablespoon extra-virgin coconut oil, at room temperature
1 teaspoon pure vanilla extract
⅛ teaspoon ground cinnamon
¼ cup garbanzo bean (chickpea) flour
1/16 teaspoon coarse sea salt or specialty salt, like pink Himalayan (optional)

Place the chocolate in a medium bowl. Add the hot water 1 tablespoon at a time, stirring until the chocolate is melted (don't use all of the water if you don't need to—stop when the chocolate is melted). Fold in the coconut oil, vanilla, and cinnamon. Then slowly stir in the garbanzo bean flour, 1 tablespoon at a time, to form a thick batter. Pinch off pieces of the batter, pat the pieces into round balls, and roll them between your palms to form 8 truffles. Place the truffles on wax paper, sprinkle each with sea salt if you like, and refrigerate them at least 15 minutes. Store extra truffles, wrapped in wax paper, in a sealable container in the refrigerator. They will keep for one week in the fridge. They also freeze well. Just defrost them on the counter for 5 to 10 minutes before enjoying.

Makes 8 truffles, or 4 servings

Cherry Coconut Pulse Pops

¼ cup banana slices
½ cup unsweetened coconut milk (the kind in the dairy case, not in a can)
2 tablespoons chia seeds
¼ cup canned white beans, drained and rinsed
1 teaspoon pure vanilla extract
¼ cup frozen cherries
¼ cup chopped dark chocolate

In a blender or food processor, combine the banana, coconut milk, chia seeds, beans, and vanilla, and blend the mixture until it is smooth. Stir in the cherries and chocolate, and spoon the mixture into 4 BPA-free pop molds. Freeze overnight. These pops will keep for two weeks in the freezer.

Makes 4 servings

Pulse Pumpkin Spice Mini Muffins

½ cup garbanzo bean (chickpea) flour
½ cup almond flour

½ cup organic cane sugar

1 teaspoon pumpkin pie spice

½ teaspoon baking soda

½ teaspoon baking powder

¼ teaspoon sea salt

½ cup extra-virgin olive oil

1 teaspoon pure vanilla extract

1 cup canned organic pumpkin

Preheat the oven to 350°F. In a large bowl, whisk together the garbanzo bean flour, almond flour, sugar, spice, baking soda, baking powder, and salt. Fold in the oil, vanilla, and pumpkin to form a smooth batter. Spoon 1 tablespoon of the batter into each of 24 paper cup–lined mini muffin cups. Bake for 15 minutes, or until a toothpick inserted into the center of a muffin comes out clean. Cool them for at least 15 minutes before enjoying.

Wrapped, these will keep for three days at room temperature. Or freeze them for up to two weeks; just defrost them at room temperature for 15 minutes before enjoying.

Makes 24 mini muffins, or 8 servings

Five More Ways to Feel Satisfied

Here are five other ways to feel like you've had plenty.

Stop and Smell the Spices

Incorporating fragrant spices into indulgences not only adds flavor and antioxidants to sweet treats, but it's also a smart weight-loss strategy. A recent Dutch study found that when volunteers could control their own dessert portions, they ate 5 to 10 percent less of the aromatic selections than the nonaromatic options. So before taking a bite of your pumpkin spice mini muffin, take a deep breath, close your eyes, and enjoy a leisurely sniff.

Don't Forego the Muffin Liners

You'll notice that in the instructions for the brownie bites and pumpkin spice mini muffins, I advise spooning the batter into paper liners rather than pouring it directly into the pan. There's an important reason for this. When you unwrap each treat, the paper acts like a mental speed bump to slow you down. Also, seeing the wrappers signals your brain to keep track of how much you've consumed. Research shows this kind of visual evidence prompts people to eat less without even trying.

Set the Mood

Soft lighting and music aren't just for romance; they can also create a mood that curbs eating, Cornell University researchers have found. Under these two conditions, restaurant diners rated their meals as more enjoyable and consumed nearly 20 percent less. Try it at home, especially when enjoying a treat.

Slow Your Pace

In our fast-paced world, it's easy to unknowingly gobble down your food. But eating too fast curtails the release of hormones that induce feelings of fullness, prompting mindless overeating, according to a study published in the *Journal of Clinical Endocrinology & Metabolism*. Another study, from the University of Rhode Island, found that compared to fast eaters, slow eaters take in about four times fewer calories per minute and feel more satisfied, even when they eat less food. To slow your pace, eat without distractions—turn off the TV, close your computer, and put away reading material. Put your utensil or food down between bites, and stop when you feel you've had just enough, even if you haven't finished all of your treat.

Recall Your Treat Time

Merely thinking about a meal you ate can prompt you to eat less later that day. That's what scientists from the University of Birmingham found when they asked volunteers to reflect on either an eating experience or a commute.

What to Do When You're Tempted to Overindulge

You might be wondering, *What if I feel like eating all of the brownie bites or other treats, rather than just one portion?*

We've all felt out of control at times, scarfing down a box of cookies when we're stressed or devouring half a chocolate cream pie for comfort when we're sad. If you have a history of emotional overeating, and you don't feel ready to incorporate dessert indulgences into your eating strategy, wait until you do.

How can you gain more control over how much you eat? Willpower—no matter how much you can muster—won't make emotional eating go away, but I believe that daily meditation, explained in chapter 7, can help tremendously.

Overcoming emotional eating is a process that involves several steps. First, you become aware of your pattern. Then you identify the emotional need that's driving you to eat, such as sadness, happiness, anger, or fear. Finally, you test out alternative behaviors that meet the emotional need, so you no longer feel drawn to use food. This process doesn't happen overnight. I liken it to learning to speak a new language: you need a great deal of awareness and practice before it starts to become second nature.

That said, one tool that can help straightaway is to choose a word or image that represents how amazing you feel when you're in balance. You might choose "free," with an image of a bird soaring, or "blossoming," with a photo of a blooming flower. This is a technique I often use with my clients. Let me give you an example of how it helps curb emotional eating.

One of my clients grew up using food as a way to bond, show love, and buffer anxiety. She rarely listened to her body's hunger cues. As a result, she struggled with her weight and constantly felt sluggish and bloated—"just blech," as she described it. When she began eating healthfully, her energy skyrocketed, her digestive health improved, she started shedding pounds, and she felt more confident at work. Still, after a bad day at the office, she'd get sucked back into making emotionally charged food choices.

When I told her about this technique, she chose the word "radiant" and an image of the sun. Then she strategically placed index cards, sticky notes, and photos at her home and office and even in her car. One day, after a tiff with her sister, she felt drawn to the kitchen, but seeing "radiant" and a glowing sunrise photo reminded her of how great she felt when she ate in a way that honored her body's needs rather than her mind's. So she called a friend, talked it out, and got through the moment.

This technique can help you stay connected to the benefits of eating in a balanced way. In the moment, when your stress level is through the roof and you feel the need to stuff down sweets, that immediate need takes precedence. You don't think about why diving into that pint of ice cream is an action you'll regret. But if you can focus on the importance of breaking your pattern, you're less likely to follow through.

I invite you to try this strategy yourself.

This exercise is also helpful if you don't have a pattern of emotional eating, but you tend to overeat simply because you're enjoying a food and don't want the experience to end. In either case, if you do end up ignoring your key word or image and eating more than you intended to, don't beat yourself up. That only leads to negative emotions, which actually fuel more emotional eating and can lead to giving up and jumping off a healthy path altogether.

STAYING CONNECTED GRID		
When I eat healthfully I feel . . . (use as many words or sentences as you'd like)	What one word sums up these feelings?	What one image represents this word?

THE POWER OF FIBER

I have devoted an entire chapter in this book, chapter 4, to the power of pulses, but a French-Swedish team recently investigated a specific component of these gems: fiber. Fiber is not digested or absorbed from the GI tract into the bloodstream. Scientists discovered that when fiber is fermented by intestinal bacteria, substances are created that regulate blood sugar, reduce sensations of hunger, and boost metabolic rate. Each recipe in this chapter includes fiber-rich pulses as well as other fiber-rich ingredients, like almond flour, dates, bananas, chia seeds, cherries, and pumpkin. So any treat you choose will deliver a formidable fiber boost!

WHAT IF I HAVE MORE OF A SALT TOOTH THAN A SWEET TOOTH?

If you don't have a sweet tooth, there's no need to incorporate any of these treats into your diet. However, if salt is more your thing, you may enjoy the truffles for two reasons. First, dark chocolate has been shown to curb cravings for both sweet and salty foods. Also, you have the option of sprinkling the truffles with $\frac{1}{16}$ teaspoon of coarse sea salt or a specialty salt, like pink Himalayan. You may be thinking, *Salt, really? In a weight-loss book?* But the amount is scant. One-sixteenth of a teaspoon provides less than 150 milligrams of sodium, and the recipe makes four servings. Yet just that pinch, bundled with the antioxidant- and mineral-rich dark chocolate and garbanzo bean flour, may completely fulfill your hankering for salt.

If chocolate just isn't your thing, some of the foods you might find most satisfying are the DIY microwave popcorn or Oven-Roasted Sweet Potato "Fries" (both on page 175), energy accessories you're able to enjoy every day. If you'd like to salt them, be sure to use a measured and minimal amount, as I did with the truffles. Too much sodium can trigger water retention and bloating, as well as thirst, which you may confuse with hunger.

WHAT IF I WANT TO INDULGE IN A DIFFERENT SWEET TREAT INSTEAD?

That's okay. I don't expect the four recipes in this chapter and three Rapid Pulse puddings to be the only treats you indulge in ever again. To learn how to incorporate other treats into my plan, see How to Squeeze In a Splurge on page 301.

WHY YOU WON'T FIND CALORIE, CARB, OR SUGAR COUNTS HERE

Sometimes people ask me for my recipes' nutrition information. Though I have excellent software for calculating this data, I don't think it's necessary. Surprised?

The truth is, the most current research indicates that not all calories are created equal, and the same applies to fat, carb, sugar, or protein grams. In other words, even if two muffins have equal calorie counts, the one made with refined white flour, refined sugar, and shortening will have a completely different effect on your blood sugar and insulin response, fullness and satiety levels, and subsequent appetite than a muffin made with bean and nut flours, fruit, coconut, and extra-virgin olive oils.

You've probably noticed this effect yourself. Surely you feel more satisfied when you've snacked on a crisp apple and a handful of almonds than when you've chosen sugary candy with the same calorie count. Nonetheless, many people insist that knowing and tracking numbers is necessary. If you're among them, revisit the remarkable studies I cited in chapter 4. These studies show that including pulses in a meal boosts postmeal fullness, suppresses hunger, reduces later snack attacks, curbs the desire to eat processed foods, enhances calorie and fat burning, and whittles waistlines.

Because certain foods affect metabolism, appetite, and weight control differently than others, getting caught up in numbers isn't necessary, and I'm sure you'll agree, letting go of numbers is quite freeing!

My Story

Kristi Fletcher, age 40

Lost 20 pounds and 11.25 inches

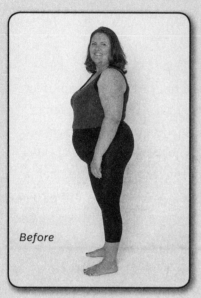

Before

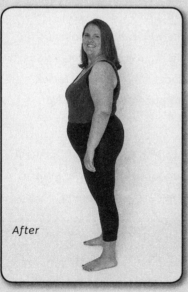

After

Before I met Cynthia I was eating terribly. I was hungry all the time, I craved sweet, then salty, then sweet again, and I drank very little water and mostly diet soda. I love healthy food, but I was being controlled by cravings and poor planning and proportions. Now I can say that I feel completely in control and confident about my eating!

I started seeing results right away, and lost 8 pounds during the Rapid Pulse! The Rapid Pulse was strict and challenging, but if I had skipped it and started with the Daily Pulse, it would have been a completely different experience. Once I started the Daily Pulse, food tasted delicious and satisfying in a way I had never experienced before. It was like my taste buds had been changed. I barely needed any salt for the food to taste delicious, and I used to season quite liberally with salt! Fresh food, lightly seasoned now tastes amazing, and I feel content after each meal. I am not obsessing over food anymore!

In just thirty days my relationship with food changed so much. In the

20 21 22 23 24 25 26 27 28 29 30 31 32 33 34 35 36 3

past, I've had a hard time limiting myself to one portion of a treat. I would take a portion, and say to myself, *okay that is all I can have,* then go back for more, sometimes two or three times. I like Cynthia's idea of building splurges into meals, but I don't crave things like I used to, and I'm reacting differently to the foods I used to eat. After three weeks of following the plan I wanted to build in a splurge, so I had some of my favorite Halloween treats—candy-corn pumpkins. They tasted fake and disgusting. Wow!! I can't believe how dramatically my taste buds have changed!

When I went out of town with my family for the weekend (I'm a mom of four), I packed food for myself. While others ate restaurant food and dessert, I wasn't even tempted. It was a victory! It's getting easier and easier in social settings to just eat differently, and I really see the results of clean eating. I love the simplicity of the wardrobe analogy and how seamlessly I have been able to adapt family favorites to fit the eating plan.

This plan also improved my mood and sleep quality. I fall asleep quickly and earlier, and I have so much more energy during the day. My husband, who has always been 100 percent supportive, is so proud of how dedicated I am to this. The way he looks at me makes me want to jump over the moon!

It's just amazing to me how satisfied I feel all the time, and I still get to enjoy excellent food with no guilt. This food is delicious! After my meals I feel full but not overly full. And if I decide to go for a walk, I like being able to add another portion or half-portion of an energy accessory. I'm listening to my body and adding accessories when needed. It just makes sense. I feel great—better than I have in a long time. And I feel motivated to be active again. I have a level of confidence in myself that I haven't felt in years.

[7]

Meditation

B ack when I combined nutrition counseling with personal training, one of my clients showed up for her training session late, looking frazzled and exhausted. I adored this client, but I immediately sensed that she didn't want to be there and was in no mood for a workout. So instead of warming her up on a treadmill, our usual routine, I grabbed a couple of yoga mats, brought her to a private room, and led her through some deep breathing, guided meditation, and stretching exercises. She was completely silent until the end of our session, then she took a deep sigh, tears welling in her eyes, and said, "Thank you, Cynthia. How did you know that was *exactly* what I needed?"

I knew because of the impact meditation has had on my own life. I'm no guru, but I have found that this simple practice—which costs nothing, can be done anywhere, and requires just minutes a day—can profoundly improve your health, both emotionally and physically. In fact, for weight loss, incorporating meditation into your life may even be more beneficial than exercise!

In this chapter I share what I believe are the most important and powerful benefits of meditation—or as I like to call it "mind massage"—for your overall health and well-being, and also for your capacity to stick with this 30-day challenge. Exercise is undoubtedly important for health and weight loss, but in my experience, meditation is a vital piece of the puzzle. That's why every day of my plan includes not only a daily pulse but also a daily meditation, even if it's just a short five minutes. I believe this daily ritual is another tool that makes my plan uniquely effective.

Meditation: It's Personal

The word *meditation* may conjure up images of people sitting cross-legged on pillows, surrounded by incense and candles, chanting mantras or repeating *"ohm."* But that's not how I experience mediation. While there are many forms of this practice, one thing I love about meditation is that the philosophy behind it is personal and nonjudgmental. In other words, there's no right or wrong way to meditate, and the goal isn't to be perfect.

The type of meditation I practice is called mindfulness meditation, which, in a nutshell, involves paying attention to the present moment. Sitting for even five minutes a day to practice mindfulness mediation can help you be more mindful as you navigate your entire day. Sometimes I meditate sitting in my desk chair or on a park bench or even on the subway. When you're "in the here and now," you aren't focused on what happened in the past, and you aren't projecting into the future. This focus on the present can considerably alleviate negative emotions, such as anger and anxiety, tied to past or future thinking.

Also, when you're really aware in the moment, you experience the present in a whole new and wonderful way. Have you ever been in a place or situation that could have been an amazing experience but you found yourself unable to enjoy it because you were either dwelling on the past or worrying about the future? Maybe you didn't fully enjoy the moment because you were stewing over an argument with your mother or because you couldn't stop thinking about a work deadline. If you start practicing mindfulness meditation, you won't repeat those scenarios. Instead, you'll truly experience each moment, whether you're taking in spectacular scenery on vacation or simply eating a meal, walking outside, petting your dog, or having a conversation with your significant other.

Later in this chapter I explain how to get started meditating, but first, let me take you through some of the incredible research findings about mindfulness mediation. Let's start with the reasons this practice will help you lose weight.

Meditation Quells Inflammation

On page 23 I explained how inflammation is tied to obesity and chronic disease. This link is one reason that antioxidants, which fight inflammation, are so important for long-term weight control and optimal health. But meditation is another way to help control inflammation, research shows.

Scientists at the University of Wisconsin–Madison compared two interventions aimed at reducing stress: the mindfulness-based stress-reduction (MBSR) approach and a program that focused on nutrition, walking, core strengthening, and music therapy. (MBSR is a behavioral medicine program created by Jon Kabat-Zinn, professor of medicine emeritus and founding director of the Stress Reduction Clinic and the Center for Mindfulness in Medicine, Health Care, and Society at the University of Massachusetts Medical School.) After eight weeks, the subjects underwent a test designed to induce psychological stress. In addition, to trigger inflammation, their skin was exposed to a cream made with capsaicin, the substance that gives hot peppers their fire. Tests that measured immune and endocrine responses were also collected. The researchers found that the mindfulness-based approach was significantly more effective at reducing stress-induced inflammation. In other words, the changes in immune and endocrine function were actually physiological, not just psychological. The upshot: mindfulness mediation can help transform your body at the cellular level, where conditions like inflammation affect your metabolism, weight, and health.

Mindfulness Lowers Stress Hormone Levels

Both physical and emotional stress trigger the adrenal gland to release a notorious hormone called cortisol. High cortisol levels have been shown to drive up appetite; increase cravings for sugary, fatty foods; and cause surplus calories to be deposited as belly fat. Controlling stress is the best way to prevent cortisol from surging, and a recent study from University of California, Davis, found that mindfulness is a particularly effective strategy. Scientists measured the mindfulness scores and cortisol levels of volunteers before and after an intensive, three-month mindfulness medi-

MINDFULNESS CAN HELP YOU ADOPT THIS EATING PLAN MORE EFFORTLESSLY

Mindfulness can improve memory, a benefit that will help you tremendously as you adopt your new approach to eating. In chapter 3, I include a handy cheat sheet to help you memorize the "diet wardrobe" framework; the quick summary will help, but daily meditation may help even more.

In a study published in *Psychological Science,* researchers randomly assigned forty-eight students to either a class that taught mindfulness or a class that covered nutrition. Shortly before the classes, the students were given tests that measured reasoning, memory, and mind wandering. A week after the classes ended, the students were tested again. Those in the mindfulness group had significantly improved both reasoning and memory. Their minds also wandered less during the postclass tests, effects that weren't seen among the students in the nutrition-only class. So as you set out to fully grasp the new approach to eating I've laid out in this book, incorporating even five minutes of meditation into each day can help you embrace it.

••

ANTI-INFLAMMATION IS KEY TO HEALTH, REGARDLESS OF WEIGHT

We've long known that chronic inflammation is linked to premature aging, type 2 diabetes, heart disease, brain disorders, and obesity, among other conditions. Now a study from University College Cork in Ireland finds that controlling inflammation protects health, regardless of weight. This finding may explain why some obese people remain healthy, even though excess weight is generally tied to an increased risk of chronic disease. In the study, researchers found that both normal-weight and obese people with low levels of inflammatory markers in their blood were metabolically healthy. The takeaway: thinness doesn't always equate to better health, and focusing on lifestyle habits that reduce inflammation, including meditation and eating anti-inflammatory plant-based foods, can help to safeguard your health, regardless of your size.

••

tation retreat. Researchers found a correlation between high mindfulness scores and low levels of cortisol, both before and after the retreat. In other words, those who were more mindful prior to the retreat already had lower levels of the stress hormone, and those whose mindfulness scores increased after the retreat also showed a decrease in cortisol. In fact, the greater the increase in mindfulness, the lower the cortisol levels.

Meditation Fights Burnout

Given the results of the stress studies I just mentioned, it's no surprise that meditation and mindfulness training have been used to reduce burnout among teachers and medical students. At the University of Wisconsin–

Madison, researchers recruited teachers to take part in the mindfulness-based stress-reduction (MBSR) course. The teachers were randomly selected to participate or not participate in guided meditation at home for at least fifteen minutes a day. They also learned specific strategies for preventing and coping with stress in the classroom. One of these strategies was "dropping in," which means briefly bringing attention to the sensation of breathing and observing thoughts and emotions. The training also included practices aimed at increasing kindness. The teachers who received the mindfulness training showed measureable reductions in psychological stress, improvements in classroom organization, and more self-perceived compassion. In comparison, those who didn't receive the eight-week training showed signs of increased stress and burnout over the school year.

In the medical world, up to 60 percent of physicians experience burnout, which can interfere with the quality of care they provide, decrease their compassion for patients, and increase their risk of making medical errors. To train doctors more effectively, Wake Forest Baptist Medical Center now provides third-year medical students with guided relaxation and mindfulness meditation training, which speaks volumes about how Western medicine now views the effectiveness of this practice.

Mindfulness Can Help Minimize Impulsive Eating

After a rough day, have you ever spotted the rack of candy at the grocery checkout and spontaneously tossed a chocolate bar onto the conveyor belt? Throughout each day, we encounter countless temptations, and these are especially strong when our emotions are triggered. But according to a study from the University of Toronto Scarborough, mindful individuals—who are adept at letting go of their feelings and thoughts rather than acting upon them—are less likely to seek immediate rewards. To test how volunteers responded to feedback on their work performance, researchers monitored brain responses as participants received reactions to their work that was positive, neutral, or negative. Researchers found that mindful individuals were significantly less responsive to reward-based feedback. This study supports the idea that mindfulness enhances self-control. Another study, from the University of Utah, found that mindful individuals have better control over their mood and behavior, leading to more emotional stability throughout the day and better quality sleep at night. These results suggest that enhancing mindfulness can help you feel less susceptible to spontaneously turning to food for emotional support.

Meditating May Help You Become More Physically Active

Though exercise has been proven to relieve stress, many of my clients skip workouts when they're stressed. This pattern is common, according to a recent Yale University report. Researchers examined numerous studies that looked at the influence of stress on physical activity. They found that, overwhelmingly, psychological stress prompted people to exercise less and engage in more sedentary behavior. The causes of stress included work-family conflicts, job strain, being a caregiver, family illnesses, and stressful life events, like final exams for college students. Because meditation has been shown to diminish stress so effectively, it may also reduce the barriers to being more active.

I know I find this to be true for myself. When I'm less consistent with my daily meditation, I see exercise, including my usually beloved walks, as a burden or just another task I don't have time for. But when I'm regularly mediating, I feel more eager to go for walks, even when I'm dealing with work or family stress. In fact, when I'm consistent with meditation, I perceive walking as a way to further de-stress, think through problems, and achieve some clarity.

Meditation Can Curb Hunger and Binge Eating and Boost Self-Esteem

Researchers at Massachusetts General Hospital enrolled overweight and obese corporate employees in a twenty-week mind–body intervention that included mindfulness mediation. The upshot: the volunteers lost, on average, nearly 10 pounds and reported less hunger, less desire to eat, and improvements in self-confidence, self-esteem, physical activity, healthy eating, and stress management. In a U.K. study, researchers examined how mindfulness affected weight loss in sixty-two women ages nineteen to sixty-four. Half the volunteers were randomly invited to attend a mindfulness workshop, and the rest were simply asked to make no changes. After six months, researchers found that the women in the mindfulness group lost 5 more pounds than those in the control group, primarily due to a reduction in binge-eating episodes. They also were more physically active than the women who didn't receive mindfulness training.

Meditation Tunes Out Distractions

Meditation helps you regulate a brain wave called the alpha rhythm, which in turn enables you to tune out agitations and diversions. This is no small benefit! In an impressive study, researchers from Massachusetts General Hospital, Harvard Medical School, and the Massachusetts Institute of Technology randomly assigned healthy meditation novices to either the eight-week mindfulness-based stress-reduction (MBSR) program or no meditation. They also measured brain activity, including alpha rhythms, before, during, and after the study period. After two months, the volunteers who completed the mindfulness training made faster and more significant adjustments to the alpha rhythm than the nonmeditators. Scientists say the study supports the notion that mindfulness meditators are better able to quickly screen out distractions.

Here's why I'm fascinated by this finding: When my clients send me their daily food diaries, the journals frequently indicate that distractions prompt them to overeat. Specifically, when my clients feel preoccupied by emotions or tasks, they often skip meals, which leads to rebound overeating or impulsively succumbing to comfort foods and treats. If my clients could sweep away those distractions even half the time, I have no doubt they would lose significantly more weight.

Meditation Relieves Food-Is-My-Friend Loneliness

When my clients fill out their food diaries, they indicate not only what and how much they ate but also how they were feeling emotionally before, during, and after eating. This additional information provides valuable insight into their relationship with food. For example, feelings of loneliness pop up often as triggers for overeating. Many clients say that foods like ice cream and baked goods soothe them or allow them to disconnect from uncomfortable emotions. Others make the connection that food keeps them company, serving as a comforting companion. If you find this to be true for you, meditation can help. One study from Carnegie Mellon University recruited forty healthy adults ages fifty-five to eighty-five who completed blood tests and measures of loneliness at the beginning and end of the study. Participants were randomly assigned to either the eight-week mindfulness-based stress-reduction (MBSR) program or no intervention. After two months, those who participated in the mindfulness program experienced a decrease in loneliness. Again, the effect wasn't just emotional; they also had reductions in blood markers for inflammation.

Meditation Helps You See Yourself More Accurately

I love that that the primary goal of mindfulness meditation is simply to be aware in the moment. After meditating, even for five minutes, try to stay focused on what you're experiencing, both physically (Do you have a headache? Does your back hurt?) and emotionally (Are you feeling sad? Are you thinking about an unresolved disagreement?). Commit to remaining neutral and nonjudgmental about what you observe. You may even silently finish the statements *I am noticing* _____ (fill in the blank), *I am thinking* _____ , *I am feeling* _____ .

One scientist at Washington University in St. Louis believes this kind of awareness can be incredibly beneficial for overcoming "blind spots"—in other words, for discovering things you may not have realized about yourself that could be impeding your ability to change. We're generally trained to focus on our own positive qualities and fend off negative feelings. But if you're able to nonjudgmentally observe your true thoughts and feelings, you may be more open to examining them without becoming defensive or critical of yourself. This knowledge can enable you to identify patterns, such as self-sabotage, that interfere with your health goals.

During one mindfulness meditation session, I observed tension in my neck and shoulders, something I hadn't been aware of. When I opened up to my thoughts, I noticed I was thinking about the chilled bottle of pinot grigio in the fridge my hubby had bought (and I prefer red!). As I allowed my feelings to surface, I realized I was angry about a situation that had happened earlier in the week, something I had been unknowingly hanging on to. Just that recognition allowed me to begin to release my pent-up emotions, and I started to feel the tension ease in my shoulders. Now calmer, I was also able to objectively revisit the incident, recognize that it wasn't really about me, and let it go. If I hadn't, I might have cracked open that bottle of wine, not to leisurely enjoy some vino but to subconsciously cope with unexpressed anger.

How to Get Started

It's difficult to describe how to meditate in writing, so I created a free five-minute guided video to get you started. Just log on to my website, www
.CynthiaSass.com, click on the "Mindful" tag at the top of the page, press
play, and follow along.

During the first week of this program, I encourage you to watch and
practice this guided meditation just once a day. Then, as it becomes part of
your normal routine, practice being mindful throughout the day on your
own. One technique I find particularly effective is something I learned in
a meditation class at UCLA called STOP, which stands for Stop, Take a
breath, Observe, Proceed. STOP is from Dr. Kabat-Zinn's mindfulness-based stress-reduction (MBSR) approach. When I catch myself feeling
frenzied, or notice my mind wandering into the past with "I wish I would
have" thoughts or propelling me into the future with "What if" worries, I imagine a big red STOP sign and put the acronym into action. In
those moments, I take a deep breath and draw my attention to the present moment, observing the sights, smells, colors, and sounds surrounding
me. When I'm experiencing those things fully in the moment, there is no
room for past or future, because they don't exist in the present, and in that
space, they disappear! If you sense past/future thoughts creeping in when
you try this technique yourself, visualize an imaginary broom sweeping
them away so you remain engaged in the now.

I know this may all sound very new age or hippie-dippie, but the science to support mindfulness meditation is solid, and on many occasions
I personally have experienced the transformative power of mindfulness.
For example, recently in New York City I was rushing around, running
errands between meetings. Stressed about all the things I had to do, I
began worrying about how I could possibly meet all of my deadlines, and
my head was pounding. As I walked past the corner of Union Square, I
noticed several people had stopped to look at a tree, and some were point-ing and taking pictures. I asked the man standing next to me what everyone

was looking at, and he said, "Up there—it's a red-tailed hawk." Suddenly I saw it, and it was majestic. The hawk's red tail reminded me to STOP, so I closed my eyes for a moment and took a deep breath. As I watched the hawk, I suddenly became aware of the breeze on my cheek, the smell of the crisp fall air, the brilliantly colored leaves on the trees and covering the grass below, and the excitement in the voices of the strangers around me, who were thrilled to spot wildlife in the city. In those moments, I was no longer thinking about work and deadlines. My whole body relaxed, and I could feel my heart rate slow down. The tension in my jaw, which was probably causing my headache, simply vanished. The hawk swooped down to catch a rat, and as everyone gasped, it flew away. As I went about my day, I almost felt like I'd hit a reset button on my emotions. Instead of being caught up in worry, I focused on what needed to be done that day, and because I was able to stay present, I felt much more engaged and confident during my afternoon meetings. My headache went away, and I woke up the next day feeling more capable of accomplishing my tasks on time.

Again, I'm not an advanced meditator, but I've practiced enough to notice how powerful mindfulness meditation can be. Here are my favorite things about this practice:

- It's all about self-discovery.
- I can progress at my own pace.
- It's not about being perfect. In fact, if I fall out of practice, I'm encouraged not to judge myself or beat myself up but rather to simply start again.
- It makes me feel more alive and connected to myself, others, and nature.
- It helps me create more balance in my life.
- It makes me feel happier!

This chapter is only a brief introduction to mindfulness mediation, and you've probably noticed that many of the studies I cited refer to eight-week classes. Right now, I just want to introduce you to the idea of meditation and get you started, but if you're interested in studying more formally, there are some great resources accessible online. I've studied meditation through several organizations in Florida and New York and most recently through UCLA's Mindful Awareness Research Center (MARC). MARC offers affordable classes online that are open to anyone. Check out their website at http://marc.ucla.edu. Another fantastic resource is the University of Massachusetts Center for Mindfulness, which offers an eight-week online mindfulness-based stress-reduction (MBSR) course. Visit www .umassmed.edu/cfm/stress-reduction-mbsr-online.

Seven Magnificent Reasons to Embrace the Present and Live a Mindful Life

Mindful Eating Reduces Belly Fat

A great deal of research has looked at using mindfulness practices before, during, and after eating. At the University of California, San Francisco, researchers found that mastering simple mindful eating techniques helped women lose weight, even without dieting. None of the women in the study were on calorie-counting or weight-loss diets. Half participated in mindfulness training, which taught them to become aware of their feelings of hunger, fullness, and satisfaction. After week six they were also asked to attend a full-day silent meditation retreat. Before and after the four-month study, researchers measured the women's psychological stress and their fat and cortisol levels. Women in the mindfulness group who were best able to use the techniques to tune in to their bodies had greater decreases in stress and cortisol levels as well as significant reductions in belly fat.

To experience mindful eating, try this exercise: Place a small portion of fruit on a plate, like a single grape or berry or a slice of banana or apple. Follow the guided meditation video on my website, then place the fruit in your mouth, close your eyes, and focus on directing all of your attention toward the eating experience. Notice the texture, flavor, aroma, temperature, the way the fruit feels in your mouth, and how your body and mind are responding. Jot down your observations. Next, try this exercise with a full meal. Commit to eating this meal seated at a table without distractions—no TV, Internet, reading, or even music. Slow your pace, putting your utensil down between bites, and remain mindful throughout the meal. If you notice distracting thoughts creeping in, use the imaginary broom to sweep them away, and tune in to the tastes and textures of the food and to how your body is responding. When you feel satisfied and full enough, stop eating, even there's still food on your plate. Write down what you noticed, and continue this exercise daily, noticing how your observations change or grow the more you practice mindful eating.

Meditation Promotes Equanimity

One of my favorite terms is *equanimity,* which essentially means a state of psychological composure and even-temperedness, even in difficult situations. I have noticed that practicing meditation helps me tremendously in my pursuit of equanimity. When I'm actively meditating, I find that I react much more calmly to day-to-day challenges, whether they're small, like being stuck in traffic, or big, like dealing with the illness of a family member. This kind of emotional stability is helpful in numerous situations, but among my clients, I find that those who are able to achieve equanimity no longer use food to cope with life's worries and demands. That alone, without any other dietary changes, can help them lose weight.

You Can Meditate Without Meditating

If you just can't get into meditating, you might try other activities that have been shown to have similar effects, including yoga, tai chi, and qi gong. These are all activities you can perform in the comfort of your own home. You can find videos to guide you on YouTube.

CONTINUED ON PAGE 230

My Story

Amy Canning, age 28

Lost 18.9 pounds and 18.75 inches

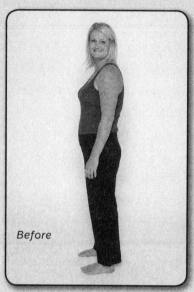

Before

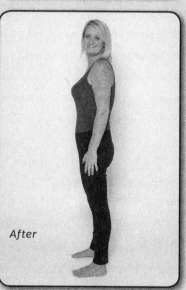

After

During the Rapid Pulse I actually thought the pudding was a sweet treat. I chose the Mango Vanilla Pulse Pudding—it tasted great, and I felt satisfied. There were a lot of temptations during the four days, but I was looking forward to seeing results and feeling more energized. Plus, I used to do diet shakes to lose weight fast, and I love the pudding soooo much more ☺ I asked if I could stick with the Rapid Pulse a little longer (the answer was no, but I could have gone at least another day).

The first day of the Daily Pulse I had trouble eating all of my breakfast—I was so full! I didn't think that would ever happen, hahaha. I literally measured everything as instructed in the recipes, and I was so scared that I gained because it seemed like so much food, but I lost more weight! I was also full of energy and didn't feel bloated. And even when I didn't sleep well I recovered quickly because my meals gave me so much energy. I could think clearly all day and felt very productive. This strategy just works for me, and I enjoy it.

20 21 22 23 24 25 26 27 28 29 30 31 32 33 34 35 36 3

Omelets with veggies and fruit on the side soon became my new favorite breakfast (I look forward to it!), and salads are an easy, fast lunch option. The plan got easier and easier every day. One day I had to eat lunch out at a pizza place. I chose to skip the pizza and eat from the salad bar (and I skipped the cheese and croutons!). I knew exactly what to choose, my salad tasted great, and I was satisfied and proud!

Throughout the thirty days I felt so confident because I knew I was getting healthier and my body was changing. My husband also lost 10 pounds by loosely following the plan with me. He was pleasantly surprised that he could lose weight while eating healthy meals that tasted great with bold flavors. Oh, and the Pulse Brownies Bites and Pulse Pumpkin Spice Mini Muffins were a hit with my whole family. I am so proud to be an encouragement to them.

This plan not only works, but it is full of good food, all while losing weight! I was a size fourteen when I started, and thirty days later I'm an eight/ten in my shorts! I woke up feeling skinnier each day, and two weeks in I was getting compliments from people who said how great I looked. They thought I was working out like crazy, and I wasn't, haha.

What surprised me the most is that I am not dependent on salt, sugar, dairy, carbs, or red meat anymore. Those were all of my staples before. Now I feel so much healthier, my skin is better, my energy level is high, I'm not as stressed, I sleep more soundly, and my stomach is no longer sensitive. Being a mommy to three kids ages four and under makes it hard to do things for me. But following this strategy is one thing I now can do for myself that makes me feel so much better.

Thank you! I feel great and love this healthy lifestyle. It has totally become a lifestyle, and I feel so proud of myself for the self-control I have over food now. I never thought I would be able to change my eating the way I have. I feel like I have discovered a whole new side to myself. I needed this really badly. I am so grateful!

Mindfulness Can Literally
Transform Your Brain

As several studies indicate, the benefits of mindfulness mediation aren't just psychological. Massachusetts General Hospital researchers used brain imaging on volunteers who took part in the eight-week mindfulness-based stress-reduction (MBSR) program. The participants, who practiced mindfulness exercises on average twenty-seven minutes a day, showed an increase in gray matter density in the brain regions associated with learning and memory, self-awareness, compassion, and introspection. They also demonstrated a decrease in gray matter density in the section of the brain tied to anxiety and stress.

Meditation Lowers Blood Pressure

Blood pressure rises in response to stress, a sensation many people experience as a rapid heartbeat, flushed face, and chest pressure. But chronically high blood pressure is often called the "silent killer" because the condition has no obvious signs. Left uncontrolled, elevated blood pressure dramatically increases the risk of stroke, heart attack, and kidney failure. That's why a recent study from Kent State University was so promising. Researchers tracked fifty-six women and men diagnosed with prehypertension—blood pressure higher than desirable, but not high enough to require medication—a condition that affects about 30 percent of Americans. Half of the patients were assigned to the eight-week mindfulness-based stress-reduction (MBSR) program. The others received lifestyle advice and engaged in muscle relaxation activities. After eight weeks, patients in the mindfulness-based intervention group had significant reductions in blood pressure measurements while the others did not. Scientists say the effects were similar to drug interventions and potentially large enough to reduce the risk of heart attack or stroke.

Meditating Each Day Keeps the Doctor Away

Because it can lower inflammation and reduce blood pressure, meditation has been used as a treatment for many conditions. Research supports the use of meditation for

- Allergies
- Anxiety
- Asthma
- Binge eating
- Cancer
- Depression
- Heart disease
- High blood pressure
- Pain
- Sleep disorders
- Substance abuse

In addition, meditation and stress reduction may help slow the progression of Alzheimer's disease and dementia, according to a pilot study led by researchers at Wake Forest Baptist Medical Center. Scientists evaluated adults ages fifty-five to ninety with mild cognitive impairment. Patients were randomized into either the eight-week mindfulness-based stress-reduction (MBSR) program or a control group that received traditional medical care. Functional MRI imaging showed that the mindfulness meditation group had significantly improved connectivity in what's known as the default mode network, the brain system that is engaged when people remember past events or envision the future. The mindfulness group also lost less matter in the brain region responsible for emotions, learning, and memory—a region known to degenerate as cognitive impairment progresses.

Meditation Helps Cultivate Compassion

In a fascinating study, scientists at Northeastern University found that meditation improves interpersonal relationships and compassion, something we could all use more of in our lives. Volunteers who completed an eight-week meditation program were compared to a control group that received no such training. One at a time, volunteers from both groups were put into a waiting room with three chairs, two filled by actors. After each participant took the last empty seat, another actor entered the room using crutches and appearing to be in a great deal of pain. The two seated actors ignored the "injured" person and continued to read or use their cell phones, creating a norm to do nothing. Among the nonmeditating participants, researchers found, only about 15 percent got up to help the injured actor, compared to 50 percent of meditators. This kind of growth in kindness and empathy, whether for a stranger in need or your own family members, friends, coworkers, or neighbors, can significantly improve your own health and happiness.

[8]

Don't Worry About Exercise—Really!

Most of my clients aren't regular exercisers. Even when they want to be and have the resources, like a home treadmill or a free gym at work or in their apartment complexes, they just aren't able to make working out a habit. When I probe a bit into their struggles, I hear three main obstacles. The first is stress. The second is lack of time—the feeling that they can't possibly fit exercise into their already jam-packed schedules. The third is a feeling that working out just isn't fun. For many of my clients, exercise feels like punishment or, at best, a chore. Instead of looking forward to breaking a sweat, they feel exercise is something they "should" do to be "good." Or it's simply penance for poor eating.

These are such high hurdles that even if I offered my clients complimentary training sessions or a free membership to a fancy health club, most of them just wouldn't be able to make it work, at least for long. I bet you're in the same boat. So, rather than include a chapter covering the health and weight-loss benefits of exercise, I'm going to help you break down this trio of barriers, so you can finally become regularly active—and actually enjoy it.

Barrier #1: Stress

One of the major goals of my daily mind massage meditation plan in chapter 7 is to reduce stress. As I explain in that chapter, stress can crush your motivation to be active and eat healthfully, or even to simply take a shower or do laundry. Some researchers actually describe stress as a "monster" because of the devastating effects it can have on your health.

Stress triggers a cascade of events in your body collectively known as the *fight-or-flight* response. It doesn't matter whether the stress is caused by an attacking dog or by financial pressures; either way, stress floods your body with hormones that spike your heart rate, breathing rate, and blood pressure, and release blood sugar to fuel your brain. At the same time, digestion and other nonessential bodily processes slow down, while your concentration and strength are revved up, priming you to respond quickly.

All of this is helpful when you're up against that attack dog or other short-term physical stresses, and when the danger is over, your body goes back to normal. But when your stress triggers are emotional and persistent, the effects linger, and the consequences can be incredibly damaging. You remain alert, but less intensely so, and as your body tries to resume its normal functions, you may experience any or all of the following side effects:

- Reduced concentration and memory
- Fatigue
- Trouble sleeping
- Elevated cortisol, a stress hormone that increases hunger and drives excess calories to be socked away as belly fat
- Excess production of stomach acid and a slowdown in digestion, leading to stomachaches and bloating

- Depression or anxiety
- Skin irritation, such as hives or eczema
- Loss of sex drive
- Dry mouth
- An increase in blood cholesterol levels
- A weakened immune system, which slows healing and makes you more vulnerable to bacterial infections and viruses

In short, when stress lingers and your body is under attack for a prolonged period of time, you're at elevated risk for disease, poor mental health, and exhaustion. This is serious stuff, and according to the American Psychological Association, 77 percent of Americans regularly struggle with the effects. Nearly half report lying awake at night due to stress, and 45 percent say stress saps their energy.

Because stress is so damaging to your body and is a major deterrent to exercise, I'm about to recommend something that may, at first, sound crazy in a weight-loss book: tell yourself you do not need to exercise to lose weight. Now, I'm not saying that physical activity isn't important; it is, for several reasons. But I don't believe that exercise, at least in the way we traditionally define it—a no pain, no gain sweatfest—is necessary for weight loss. This idea may sound radical, but it's supported by research. Are you feeling less stressed? I hope so!

Hard-core exercise often backfires, studies suggest, because people who engage in strenuous activity tend to overindulge in food and remain fairly inactive when they aren't exercising. Subconsciously, they may "reward" themselves for their hard work with behaviors that actually undermine that work.

Consider what happened when Texas Tech researchers followed 148 adults for the six weeks between Thanksgiving and New Year's Day. Half of the subjects were inactive, and half were regular exercisers who worked out about five hours a week. Over the holiday season, the exercisers and couch potatoes gained the same amount of weight, on average 2 pounds for men and about a pound for the women. The researchers aren't sure why exercise made no impact, but they suspect it's because the exercisers compensated for the extra calorie burn by eating more and moving less than usual when they weren't exercising. This phenomenon has been documented in plenty of other research.

For example, French scientists found that obese teens were less active in the hours following high-intensity exercise than in the hours following low-intensity exercise or no exercise. Another study, in older adults, found that while exercise improved heart health, exercisers didn't burn more daily calories, because they moved less than usual during the remainder of the day.

The intensity of exercise may also play a role in how you unknowingly compensate. In a study published in the *American Journal of Clinical Nutrition,* University of Ottawa researchers divided moderately active women into three groups. One group didn't exercise, another burned 350 calories per session through low-intensity exercise, and the third group burned 350 calories through high-intensity exercise. The high-intensity exercisers ate more at their postworkout meal than did both the low-intensity exercisers and the inactive group. The researcher concluded that increasing exercise intensity subconsciously triggers a compensatory increase in calorie intake.

Over the years I've seen numerous men and women attempt to lose weight through hard-core exercise, like training for a marathon or putting in countless hours at the gym, only to remain exactly the same size. So though it may seem counterintuitive, when it comes to exercise and weight loss, less is actually better than more!

One of the most compelling studies illustrating this point comes from the University of Copenhagen. Scientists assigned sixty-one inactive, moderately overweight men to one of three groups. One remained sedentary, one exercised moderately for thirty minutes a day, and the third exercised vigorously for an hour a day. For thirteen weeks, the men kept food diaries and periodically wore motion sensors to track their daily activities apart from exercise. At the end of the study, the inactive men remained the same weight. The high-intensity exercisers lost on average 5 pounds, 20 percent less than anticipated based on the number of calories they burned working out. The men in the moderate group lost the most weight, on average 7 pounds, a whopping 83 percent *more* than what the researchers expected based on the number of calories they expended exercising. The participants' food journals and activity monitors were telling. The intense exercisers ate more than the other two groups, became couch potatoes when not exercising, and described their workouts as monotonous and exhausting. In contrast, the moderate exercisers didn't gobble down more food than at baseline, and they spontaneously became more active than before the study throughout the day. This bunch reported having higher energy levels than the men who worked out for an hour. They also reporting having more motivation and, as a result, began doing things like taking the stairs instead of the elevator or riding their bikes to work.

What I'm getting at is that pushing yourself to "make your fat cry" often backfires. After a tough workout, many of my clients feel like they've earned the right to splurge. But this mentality makes it incredibly easy to "eat back" all the calories you've burned, or more, essentially cancelling out the weight-loss effects of your workout. For example, in a one-hour circuit-training class, an average woman burns about 550 calories. But even if 100 percent of what you worked off was body fat, which is impossible, that's only enough to shrink your shape by one-seventh of a pound. Treating yourself to a chocolate pastry and a medium latte, or a large frozen yogurt with candy toppings, wipes out your ability to rely on exercise as a method of losing weight. In my experience, when you start seeing physical activity as a way of having fun rather than as a war on your thighs, this kind of game playing goes by the wayside. You no longer feel physically or emotionally triggered to compensate for making yourself miserable!

So, right now, this minute, tell yourself that letting go of exercise as a means of manipulating your body is a smart strategy for losing weight. Go ahead! Sure, your stress won't instantly vanish, but I hope you'll stop beating yourself up about not exercising as often or as hard as you think you should. The solutions in the rest of this chapter will further reduce your stress. You'll reap the rewards of moving more without suffering from the unwanted side effects tied to thinking of exercise as a punishment.

Barrier #2: Time Constraints

When I talk to my clients about the barriers to being active, the second big-gie is "I don't have time!" When this is the case, the best solution is to find an activity you enjoy that involves movement and make it part of your daily "me time."

Even my busiest clients manage to fit in some "me time" activity that helps them get through the day. It could be chitchatting with a coworker in the break room, talking on the phone, surfing the web, or catching up on celebrity gossip. Usually these breaks are brief, but they're important, because they serve as what I call "valve openers"—ways to let off steam.

Imagine a rubber band stretching to the point of snapping, a balloon filling with air until it bursts, or a simmering pot of water that's about to boil over. Each is like stress in that the pressure will eventually hit a break-ing point unless there's some kind of intervention to dial it back. On a day-to-day basis, mini "me time" breaks do the job for many of my clients. Without these breaks, stress builds to the point where the only relief is overeating, drinking too much alcohol, or both. So a seemingly frivolous diversion, like finding out which celeb couple just called it quits, actually serves an important purpose.

Right now, take a few minutes to identify your daily valve openers. Indi-cate when you tend to take these mini breaks, with whom, and how long they last. Don't judge yourself! This exercise isn't meant to make you feel guilty about sneaking in this "me time." As I've pointed out, diversions are a good thing. The purpose of this list is simply to identify how you escape. Scan through your usual day, almost like you're playing back a recording of yourself, and jot down what you discover:

_____

_____

_____

_____

_____

_____

_____

Now that you know where and how you take mini breaks, set a goal of swapping at least one break each day with an activity that involves moving your body. Just be sure to choose an activity that you'll enjoy and look forward to. That's where breaking down barrier #3 comes in. So before you finalize your swap-out plan, read the next section. Here, I help you find activities that won't make you feel like you're adding yet another miserable task to your never-ending to-do list.

Barrier #3:
The Feeling That Exercise Isn't Fun

My husband enjoys the elliptical machine. He can pop in his earbuds and happily keep pace while silently singing along to tunes on his iPod. Personally, I would rather go to the dentist than have to spend more than five minutes on that piece of equipment! And unless I'm watching a TV show I enjoy, I can't stand being on the treadmill for more than ten minutes. Apart from being incredibly boring, these kinds of exercises strike me as toil, and before too long, every minute feels like torture.

On the other hand, walking outdoors, taking in the sights, feeling the breeze on my face and sun on my back—now, that's a different story. Outdoors I can walk and walk and walk without feeling like I'm "exercising," because it just feels natural and enjoyable. But this is only the case when I'm not equating walking with working out. The minute I find myself feeling like I "should" go for a walk, I get turned off; the exact same activity morphs from something I enjoy into something that feels obligatory and is tied to judgment (I'm "good" if I do it and "bad" if I don't). Suddenly,

I'm feeling resentful, anxious, and rebellious. Sound familiar? Overcoming this negative association may just be the most important way to stop avoiding physical activity and finally become regularly active.

To get started, list every form of exercise you loathe. Include every activity you've tried in the past or have even engaged in regularly that has triggered feelings of negativity or resentment:

_____

_____

_____

_____

_____

_____

Now vow never to engage in these activities again! (As long as they still make you feel this way, of course.) Exercising in ways that don't feel good—even if they're "good for you"—will backfire. You'll either burn out and quit or, like the volunteers in the studies I cited previously, compensate by eating or resting more. Either way, you won't lose weight.

Now the fun part: finding truly enjoyable activities that involve moving your body. Really take time to think this through. Below, list every activity you relish that requires movement—activities you would enjoy even if they didn't burn a single calorie. For example, in addition to walking and hiking, my favorite ways to be active, I really enjoy dancing, swimming, roller-skating, cross-country skiing, biking, and skipping rope. I also love fun noncompetitive sports, like beach volleyball, tennis, table tennis, and shooting hoops (just making baskets, not really playing basketball). List what comes to mind for you.

_____

_____

_____

_____

_____

_____

_____

_____

Now list activities you've always wanted to try but haven't yet tried. My list includes kayaking, surfing, racquetball, skateboarding, and jumping on a trampoline.

_____

_____

_____

_____

_____

_____

When you visualize yourself engaging in the "fun" activities on your list, how do you feel? My guess is words like *carefree* and *I feel like a kid again* come to mind, and these positive thoughts create an important domino effect. When you're moving your body in ways that are amusing, you feel happier. The fact that you're also burning calories becomes icing on the cake. Helping you cultivate play through movement is one of my goals in this chapter.

Not surprisingly, much of the research on play is focused on children. However, one recent study in older adults found that those who are more playful also are more optimistic, cheerful, positive, enthusiastic, relaxed, spontaneous, and creative. These traits foster positive emotions that support balanced emotional health and enhance resilience to hardship. Making movement enjoyable not only breaks down the "boredom" barrier to being active but also helps dismantle one of the other significant barriers: chronic stress.

Next, build the activities you enjoy into your day, using the following five steps:

Step 1

Choose one activity from your fun list, and commit to replacing one of your "me time" activities with this form of movement.

Let's say surfing the web is one of your favorite diversions, and dancing is one of your fun movements. Bookmark the YouTube video of your favorite danceable song, and use your web time to dance all the way through it.

Whatever you choose, commit to making the switch once a day. In fact, take a moment to write down your first swap:

I will trade (usual "me time" activity) _____

_____

for (fun movement activity) _____

_____.

Step 2

Trade some food prep time for movement time.

There are only so many hours in the day, so to carve out time to be more active, you'll likely have to shave time from another activity, perhaps food prep. A recent study from Ohio State University found that for every additional ten minutes a day adults spent on food preparation, they were less likely to exercise for ten minutes. The findings applied equally to men and women, to single and married adults, and to parents and people who don't have children. The good news is, if you take ten minutes away from food prep, you can still enjoy healthy meals that support my plan. (You'll find fast meal options and grab-and-go choices throughout chapter 5.)

One fantastic way to spend some of the time you saved on meal prep is to take a fifteen-minute stroll after each meal. This habit can help normalize blood sugar levels for up to three hours after eating, according to a study from George Washington University, and may cut your risk of developing type 2 diabetes more effectively than taking one continuous forty-five-minute walk. In the study, researchers recruited healthy adults at risk of developing type 2 diabetes due to inactivity and high fasting blood sugar levels. Scientists found that incorporating three daily fifteen-minute postmeal walks at an easy-to-moderate pace was as effective as taking one daily forty-five-minute walk for regulating blood sugar over a twenty-four-hour period. Even better, the postmeal walks were more effective at normalizing blood sugar after meals, the riskiest time for prediabetics, when blood sugar levels spike the most. Even if you can't squeeze in a walk after every meal, commit to doing this once a day. Or trade some of your food prep time for one of the fun activities on your list.

Step 3

Combine social time with movement time.

Some of your daily downtime is likely spent socially, with coworkers, friends, or family members. Ask some of the significant people in your life to spend your time together moving. You could go for a walk to catch up rather than chatting over a cup of tea. Or you could recruit your significant other, daughter, or roommate to dance with you every day, or try out a new activity together. A few examples include watching a Bollywood video, music video, or a clip from a musical with a dance sequence (like *Grease, West Side Story, Saturday Night Fever,* or *Slumdog Millionaire*) and learning the moves side by side.

When my clients examine how they spend their social time, they find it typically revolves around either being inactive, eating, or both. Switch it up. You'll still enjoy quality time with the people you care about, and moving in fun ways together can breathe new life into your relationships. Take a minute to write down a few people you'd like to approach with this idea. Include the activities you two might enjoy doing together.

I'll ask _____

to (fun movement activity) _____

instead of (the usual way we spend time together) _____

_____.

I'll ask _____

to (fun movement activity) _____

instead of (the usual way we spend time together) _____

_____.

I'll ask _____

to (fun movement activity) _____

instead of (the usual way we spend time together) _____

_____.

Step 4

Make movement plans for the weekend.

Traditional exercise advice has advocated working out five to six times a week, but newer research suggests that weekend-only exercisers can be just as healthy as those who exercise daily.

Scientists at Queen's University in Ontario studied over two thousand adults to determine if exercise frequency affected their risk of being diagnosed with metabolic syndrome. This syndrome is a cluster of risk factors that raise the chances of developing heart disease, type 2 diabetes, and stroke. To be diagnosed with metabolic syndrome, you must have at least three of five conditions: a large waistline (over 35 inches for women and over 40 inches for men); high blood pressure (130/85 or higher); high triglycerides (150 or above); low "good" HDL cholesterol (less than 40 for men and less than 50 for women); and high fasting blood sugar (100 or higher).

SEX COUNTS AS PHYSICAL ACTIVITY!

According to a recent study published in the *New England Journal of Medicine,* the energy expended during sex is on par with walking at about 2.5 miles per hour. This means the average American woman will burn three times more calories having sex than watching TV.

Researchers found that weekend-only exercisers weren't more prone to metabolic syndrome as long as they accumulated at least 150 minutes of moderate-to-vigorous physical activity, the current weekly target from the World Health Organization. I know that racking up 150 minutes in just two days may seem like a lot, but it's easily doable with a leisurely hike, long bike ride, or active family day at a park or beach.

To put this study's conclusion into action, think of activities you enjoy that include both aerobic exercise (getting your heart rate up) and muscle resistance (using your muscles to push or pull against resistance, such as a free weight, stretchy band, or your own body weight). For example, some of my clients like to exercise while watching a favorite TV show, and they might alternate between marching in place and using handheld free weights. Exercise boosts blood flow and circulation and triggers the release of feel-good hormones, so I'm not surprised clients have told me they enjoy viewing exciting or suspenseful TV shows even more when they watch them while being active.

Step 5

Work up to 150 minutes a week.

As I've explained, the total amount of time you accumulate being active is more important than the frequency, with the goal being at least 150 minutes each week. If you've been inactive, working up to that target may seem daunting, but just take it one day at a time. Stay focused on building in

EVEN ONE DAY OF ACTIVITY CAN PROTECT YOUR HEALTH

If Saturdays and Sundays are the two days you have extra downtime, being active on even one of those days can be beneficial, according to research from University of Alabama at Birmingham. In the study, scientists recruited sixty-three women over age sixty, who performed a combination of aerobic and resistance exercises for sixteen weeks. One group exercised just once a week, a second twice a week, and a third group exercised three times per week. All three groups improved their muscle strength, cardiovascular fitness, and ability to perform everyday tasks, such as climbing stairs. And to the scientists' surprise, the benefits were identical, regardless of the exercise frequency. Though none of the women lost weight—weight loss wasn't one of the goals of the study— the increase in lean muscle mass and subsequent boost in metabolism could enhance weight loss if combined with the right eating plan.

activities you enjoy and those that don't feel like exercise, such as taking the stairs instead of the elevator or walking rather than driving to the post office.

Day to day, you may be surprised by just how many movement minutes you rack up. Use the following chart to record the number of minutes you spent being active within each hour. For example, if you walked the dog for ten minutes between 7 A.M. and 8 A.M. and you squeezed in a fifteen-minute postbreakfast walk in the same hour, record both activities and the time spent doing them in the 7-to-8 A.M. box. At the end of each day, tally your movement minutes. As the week goes on, aim to gradually increase the total. If you don't hit 150 by the end of the week, shoot for close to that goal the following week.

	MON	TUE	WED	THU	FRI	SAT	SUN
5–6 A.M.							
6–7 A.M.							
7–8 A.M.							
8–9 A.M.							
9–10 A.M.							
10–11 A.M.							
11 A.M.–12 P.M.							
12–1 P.M.							
1–2 P.M.							
2–3 P.M.							
3–4 P.M.							
4–5 P.M.							
5–6 P.M.							
6–7 P.M.							
7–8 P.M.							
8–9 P.M.							
9–10 P.M.							
10–11 P.M.							
11 P.M.–12 A.M.							
12–1 A.M.							
1–2 A.M.							
2–3 A.M.							
3–4 A.M.							
4–5 A.M.							
DAILY TOTALS							
WEEKLY TOTAL							

At this point, the big question on your mind may be, *Will all of this focus on just moving more and not "exercising" really help me lose weight?* The answer is yes!

Now, I'm not suggesting that if you're already regularly active you should stop. Nor am I suggesting you wouldn't get better results by engaging in cardio exercise five times a week and strength training twice a week. Chances are you would. But most of the people I counsel aren't regularly active, so what they really need is a way to overcome the barriers to moving more and strategies to help them consistently rack up move-ment minutes. The steps above can help you do just that, and as a result, you'll lose weight.

When you free yourself from the I-must-exercise-to-lose-weight imper-ative, you naturally feel more motivated to be active in other ways, just like the men in the University of Copenhagen study. After breaking the restrictive exercise chains, many of my clients will, without even think-ing about it, walk to a meeting rather than take a cab. Or they'll recall, "Oh yeah, I forgot—I did spend about an hour working on the lawn." They also tend to do these things more consistently, which is key to losing weight and keeping it off.

PLAN YOUR DIGITAL DETOX (OR AT LEAST YOUR DIGITAL BOUNDARIES!)

When I talk with my clients about their difficulties finding time to be active or prepare healthy meals, one issue surfaces often: overuse of their smartphones. Our phones have become a major time suck, and most of that time is spent in ways that don't feel rewarding. One client noted that every time her Facebook app notifies her that one of her "friends" has posted something—vacation photos, news of an award their child received, you name it—she feels obligated to comment. "I feel rude not acknowledging them," she told me. Others feel compelled to "keep up" on social media, repinning pins on Pinterest, uploading photos on Instagram, and tweeting their whereabouts on Twitter.

For some, social media sites can serve as an escape or a way to receive much-needed support. But for most of us, they feel like yet another chore, something we "should" be doing that isn't really benefiting us or enriching our lives. If that's the case for you, consider deleting some of your accounts or placing limits on how often you engage with them. For example, one of my clients decided to uninstall her Facebook app, unfriend anyone she didn't know personally, and limit her Facebook time to fifteen minutes each morning, mostly to send birthday wishes or check in with friends and relatives who live in other cities. The sense of freedom she felt by making this change reduced her stress level and helped her feel empowered to make other changes in her life, with the goal of creating more balance.

MY FAVORITE NEW TREND: EARTHING

Can you remember the last time you really touched nature? The last time you climbed a tree, scrambled up rocks, or walked barefoot in the grass or on the beach? Proponents of a movement called "earthing" or "grounding" believe that our modern lives separate us from direct contact with the earth, and that reconnecting with nature physically can provide important health benefits. The merits of this practice—stress reduction, better sleep, stronger immunity, and less pain—are actually backed by research. Try it yourself. Spend some of your movement minutes or meditation time outdoors, touching the earth, and take note of how the connection makes you feel.

NONEXERCISE ACTIVITY IMPROVES LONGEVITY

I've made the case that abandoning hard-core exercise supports weight loss; now let's look at the flip side: how adding physical activities can improve health. A large, twelve-year Swedish study found that no matter how much or how little subjects exercised, those who did more nonexercise physical activity, such as lawn care, gardening, fishing, and household chores, were in better health. On average, they had smaller waist measurements, higher levels of "good" HDL cholesterol, and a lower risk of poor metabolic health, which includes parameters like blood sugar and blood pressure. In addition, more exercise-free physical activity was associated with a lower risk of heart disease and a longer life span. Compared with the least active subjects, those who were most active, irrespective of regular formal exercise, had a 27 percent lower risk of heart attack or stroke and a 30 percent reduced risk of premature death from all causes.

GRATITUDE IMPROVES HAPPINESS

Researchers from the University of California, Davis, and the University of Miami conducted three experiments over ten weeks that explored the connection between gratitude and happiness. One group was asked to write down five things they were grateful for that had occurred within the last week. The second group was asked to write down five hassles they struggled with each week. The third group listed five events that took place within each week but were asked not to focus on the positive or negative aspects of these events. Those who recorded what they were grateful for experienced a 25 percent increase in happiness compared to an assessment conducted before the study. In addition, compared to the volunteers who recorded hassles or events, the gratitude trackers felt better about their lives, were more optimistic about the future, and engaged in about one and a half additional hours of exercise each week.

TRYING TO BE HAPPIER CAN MAKE YOU HAPPIER!

In a study published in the *Journal of Positive Psychology,* researchers asked two sets of volunteers to listen to upbeat music over a two-week period. One group was asked to actively try to feel happier while listening; the other group was given no such instructions. The directive made a difference: those instructed to focus on increasing their happiness experienced a greater boost in happiness compared to those who were simply asked to focus on the music.

[9]

Frequently Asked Questions About My Plan

In chapters 3 and 5 you'll find all the details you need to follow my eating plan successfully. But from time to time, my clients have raised questions that don't fit neatly into those chapters, so I've addressed them here. If you still have questions after reading this chapter, please visit my website, www.CynthiaSass.com, or reach out to me through social media via Twitter @CynthiaSass or Facebook.com/CynthiaSassFans. I'm happy to reply to your questions, offer support, and help you connect with others who are following the plan. I'd also love to hear about your favorite recipes, DIY meal creations, and results!

Weight-Loss Questions

What if I'm not losing weight?

First, it's always important to check with your doctor before starting any weight-loss program, to be sure that he or she feels it's right for you. If you have any medical conditions that need to be managed with a special diet, you may need to consult with a registered dietitian, who can create a personalized plan for your body's needs.

But what if you're a healthy adult and you're not losing weight with this plan? Start by revisiting the My Energy Needs quiz on page 87. The results of the quiz may help you adjust the plan so that you do lose weight. Also, pay close attention to the section following that quiz titled Two Additional Accessory Rules. Here I provide more suggestions for fine-tuning your portions. To optimize your metabolism, you may need to scale back or actually eat more. Believe it or not, eating too little can slow your metabolism and stall weight loss. Also, as I note in that section, listening to your body is key. As you become more familiar with your hunger and fullness patterns, energy level, and results, you will instinctively know when to scale back or when to add portions to meals.

I'm losing 1 to 2 pounds a week. Is that fast enough?

Yes! This rate of weight loss is absolutely fine, especially as you get closer to your ideal, healthy weight. In magazine stories and on TV, you may hear about people losing several pounds a week, but in reality, for many people, it's impossible to lose more than 2 pounds of body fat in one week without also losing muscle or lean tissue. Losing 2 pounds a week is actually quite a lot! It's like melting two 16-ounce tubs of shortening or eight sticks of butter from your body. As you can imagine, that kind of loss can dramatically improve how your body looks on the outside and operates on the inside.

Why is it so hard to lose weight at a faster pace? Well, consider that to lose just 1 pound of fat, you have to create a deficit of about 3,500 calories;

in other words, you need to burn about 3,500 more calories than you eat. So, to shed 1 pound of body fat in a week, you need to burn off 500 more calories each day than you consume every day for seven days. The trick is, you also need to eat enough to maintain your metabolism and support your ideal weight. If you cut your intake too much, or if you eat too little and exercise, you can wind up losing muscle tissue, slowing your metabolism, and compromising your health. Your body will switch into survival mode because it's not getting the energy and nourishment it needs to fuel your active cells and heal and replace bone, muscle, and other tissue.

In a nutshell, as you approach your weight goal, it's nearly impossible to create the kind of calorie deficit needed to lose body fat without also compromising the lean cells you need to keep. So if you're frustrated with your rate of weight loss, remember that at a slower pace, you're shrinking your fat cells while nourishing and healing the cells that keep you healthy, strong, and fit. Patience pays off! Focus on how fantastic you feel, how well your clothes fit, and the benefits beyond weight loss, like clearer skin, less facial puffiness, better sleep, and more energy.

Why does my weight fluctuate?

I know it's frustrating, but weight shifts from day to day, even hour to hour, are normal. When you weigh in, you're measuring everything that has weight—not just your muscle, bone, and body fat but also water volume (which can change quickly and wildly), undigested food (even if it will all later be burned off), and waste in your GI tract that your body hasn't eliminated yet. So if you're retaining water, your weight on the scale will be higher than it otherwise would be, even if you've lost body fat. What's important is understanding your personal patterns. Nearly all of my premenopausal clients experience water retention and bloating one week a month, and it subsides after menstruation.

Many people also experience a short-lived spike in weight after eating a meal that's saltier or higher in carbs than usual. Don't worry about these temporary, predictable fluctuations. However, if you see a steady increase in your weight, rather than an up-and-down pattern, or if you're growing out of your clothes, take an objective look at your eating habits. Have you been going out to dinner more often, eating because of stress, or indulging in treats more than a few times a week? If so, the solution to getting back on a losing track will lie in resolving these issues.

I was losing weight but then stopped. What can I do?

Check the My Energy Needs quiz on page 87 to see if your score has changed. If not, some small tweaks to the plan may help you break a plateau. For example, it may help to increase your fiber intake by choosing veggies, fruits, and whole grains that are higher in fiber. Cup for cup, black beans pack about 2.5 more grams of fiber than chickpeas, and barley provides 3 grams of fiber per ½ cup, compared to less than 2 grams in ½ cup of brown rice.

Drinking more water may also help, since water is essential for burning calories, and it helps flush out any excess sodium and fluid you may be hanging on to. Also, if you've been eating relatively dense whole grains, like whole-grain bread, pasta, and crackers, swapping these for fluffy, unprocessed whole grains, like quinoa, barley, wild rice, and popcorn, may break the plateau. Finally, meditation or other stress management tactics, along with getting more sleep, can get you back on a losing path, since both stress and a lack of sleep have been shown to interfere with weight loss. If you haven't been consistent with daily meditation, make it a priority.

I heard that drinking a tall glass of very cold ice water first thing in the morning will help me lose weight. Is this true?

While I think it's perfectly okay to do this, I don't think it's a necessity. An A.M. glass of ice water may help increase your water intake for the day, and over time, drinking more water can help you lose weight. However, the benefits of a morning glass of ice water have little to do with either drinking water first thing in the morning or the water being cold. The theory is that drinking ice-cold water revs up metabolism because your body has to burn calories to "warm up" the water. But the effect is minimal, likely less than 10 calories per cup.

However, drinking water in general has been tied to weight control. One study found that adults who drank 2 cups of water before meals shed about 40 percent more weight over twelve weeks than a second group of dieters who followed the same eating plan but didn't drink water before meals. The same group of scientists had previously found that study subjects who drank 2 cups of water before meals naturally consumed 75 to 90 fewer calories than subjects who didn't drink water before eating, enough to make a real difference over the course of several days or weeks. And water is an essential part of the calorie-burning process. In fact, some research has shown that water in general revs up metabolism, but the effect is still less than 100 calories per day from drinking 2 liters of water. Bottom line: water is great for you for lots of reasons, and I recommend aiming for 16 ounces four times a day. If you'd like to make one of those glasses ice cold and drink it first thing in the morning, that's A-OK.

I tend to nibble all day. How can I stop?

The answer depends on why you formed this habit. Do you find yourself grazing because you're physically hungry (your stomach is growling), because you're bored or feeling another emotion, or simply because food is there? The first step toward breaking an oversnacking habit is to identify your triggers. I highly recommend keeping a food diary, even for just three days, to track what and how much you eat as well as when, where, and with whom you eat. I also suggest tracking your hunger or fullness level and your mood before and after eating.

A food journal can help you detect patterns you may not be aware of. For example, it could be that you snack to put off doing work or to cope with stress. Maybe you always snack with a coworker as a way to spend time together. Or you might be in the habit of snacking while you watch TV, whether you're hungry or not. Once you understand your patterns, you can begin to consciously change them and establish a consistent eating schedule. Let's say you've recognized that you snack as a way to socialize. To break this routine, drink a mug of tea or a glass of water while you catch up with friends. Or if you snack due to anxiety, test out other ways to de-stress, like calling a friend or journaling. Awareness is the most powerful way to change any behavior.

How can I avoid tempting foods?

One excellent strategy, which I introduced on page 40, is to visualize yourself in the future. When you feel drawn toward unhealthy foods, imagine yourself a week or six months from now in a healthier, more fit body, doing something you love. Staying strongly connected to this image of yourself can help you make choices that support your ideal future outcome. When I do this exercise with my clients, and they imagine themselves interacting with family members or coworkers, cooking a healthy dinner, or going for a walk, their body language changes and their mood shifts. Quickly, they go from feeling overwhelmed to feeling excited. Some will even say, "Yes, I want that life!" Research suggests that visualizing your future self in a positive way can help you follow through with healthy behaviors.

When you feel tempted to eat because you're feeling sad or angry, test out coping strategies that don't involve food. Even if alternative activities don't feel quite as satisfying as eating, they may feel gratifying enough to help you get through a difficult moment. Sometimes you may need to express an emotion, like listening to a sad song to help you cry when you need to let it out. In other instances, you may need to distract yourself from an emotion, perhaps by keeping your mind and hands occupied with drawing or craft work. Once you find ways to meet your emotional needs or reduce the intensity of your feelings, you may no longer feel drawn toward food.

I tend to treat myself after hard workouts, and I think it's preventing me from losing weight. What can I do?

Think of it this way: Working out and then indulging is like earning $100 and then spending $100, or more. Yes, you're earning, but if you're spending at the same rate or greater, you'll never get ahead. Or, to use another analogy, exercising and then treating yourself is like paying down your credit balance, then going on a shopping spree. Sure, there is room for occasional splurging as you lose weight, but you don't want to take one step forward and two steps back. For details on how to tweak the plan if you're more active, see page 91. And for a splurge strategy that won't compromise your results, see page 301.

I've heard that not getting enough sleep can prevent weight loss. Is that true?

Yes. Sleep deprivation has been shown to spike hunger hormones, increase inflammation, and increase the risk of obesity. A lack of nightly Zs also diminishes emotional well-being, mental sharpness, productivity, and performance while increasing the risk for depression, type 2 diabetes, and heart disease. One recent study found that people who slept less than six and a half hours a night had higher body fat percentages, on average, than people who slept between eight and eight and a half hours. Another study concluded that just one sleepless night significantly increased the subjects' desire to eat starchy, fatty foods, like donuts and pizza. The effect wasn't just psychological. Researchers conducted brain scans and found that sleep deprivation changed the region of the brain responsible for food choices. So, yes, if you're struggling with your appetite or aren't seeing the results you expected, look at your sleeping habits.

What should I do if I overeat or get off track?

Don't panic, and please, please don't beat yourself up! Anxiety and critical self-talk can be self-defeating, or at the very least make it more difficult to get back on a healthy path. First, commit to the daily meditation exercise in chapter 7. Also, reestablish a regular eating schedule, and get back to drinking plenty of H_2O. Water will help flush out excess sodium, reduce water retention, and get your GI tract moving to alleviate bloat. Revisit chapter 8 to find ways to build activity into each day that you'll look forward to and enjoy. Finally, remember that this process isn't about being perfect. Your weight is a side effect of your relationship with food, and as with any relationship, you're going to have some challenging days.

But when you develop a consistent eating pattern focused on balance, nourishment, and optimal health, as this plan provides, weight loss will follow. Even better, you'll be able keep the weight off for good. So don't let one "off" meal or day derail you.

I have trouble sticking with any plan longer than a week. How can I stay motivated?

My question for you: What tends to make you lose sight of your goals or forget the reason you started this plan? Stress? Time constraints? Social obligations? Identify your barriers so you can put preventive solutions in place. For example, if you find you're running out of time to assemble meals, select meals from chapter 5 that I've identified as *Quick! Make Ahead,* or *Freeze & Reheat.* Or check out the restaurant options starting on page 172. When I'm in a hurry and don't have time to cook, I often rely on Chipotle for a go-to meal. If your eating plans go awry in social situations, suggest ways to spend time with your friends that don't revolve around eating and drinking. Or propose restaurants that you know offer menu items that fit this plan, and offer to be the designated driver if you don't want to drink. If stress is your biggest issue, revisit chapter 7 to learn about how just minutes of daily meditation can reduce stress and anxiety.

It's normal to have days when you feel like giving up. On these days, reach out to your supportive friends, focus on the rewards of staying on track that go beyond weight loss (like more self-confidence), and remember how great you feel when you're taking care of yourself. In my experience, quality-of-life benefits are the greatest motivators. Though most people who are trying to lose weight are motivated by the prospect of becoming a smaller size, I have found that on tough days, the rewards that help my clients really hang in there have to do with feeling better, both physically and emotionally. These rewards can be far more inspiring than the numbers on the scale.

Is it okay to not weigh myself?

Absolutely! In fact, it may even be healthier for you to throw away your scale. In one recent survey from the United Kingdom, women reported that what they feared most, besides visiting the dentist, was weighing in after the holidays. Stepping on a scale was even more anxiety provoking than getting dumped by a significant other or being seen naked by a colleague! In my practice, I have found that for some clients, weigh-ins are very matter-of-fact. They see the scale as a simple reality check, much like reviewing a bank statement. But for others, being weighed, even by themselves in private, can be torture. And if the number isn't what they want to see, they become consumed with anger, self-doubt, or judgment, which leads to emotional eating or giving up on healthy goals altogether. If it feels like I'm talking about you, it's okay to banish the scale. Instead, measure your progress by the way your clothes are loosening up and how you feel.

If you need a more concrete measuring stick, choose a pair of form-fitting pants and monitor how they fit. I often tell my clients that the number on the scale doesn't tell you much about your body composition. Five different women of the same height and weight can each wear different sizes, and a sixth, who weighs more, can have a lower body-fat percentage than her lighter cohorts. It's a myth that muscle weighs more than fat, because a pound of muscle and a pound of fat both weigh a pound. But dropping a pound of fat and gaining a pound of muscle can have a huge impact on how your body looks, without changing the weight on your scale at all. Just visualize a 16-ounce ultralean steak compared to a pound of lard!

One of my clients was living in scale hell. She weighed herself several times a day and was obsessed with getting to a certain number. She finally stopped when she realized she looked more toned and wore smaller jeans when her weight was actually higher than her magic target. In trying to reach a lower number, she wound up losing muscle, which slowed her metabolism. Meanwhile, the stress of pursuing a weight-focused goal increased her stress level and lowered her sleep quality. As a result, she struggled with perpetual cravings and developed a belly roll, common side effects of a spike in the stress hormone cortisol. Ditching the scale and instead focusing on how her body looked and felt was freeing; it also helped her become fitter and maintain a smaller size.

Questions About the Plan

How can I incorporate juicing into this plan?

If you'd rather juice the produce servings that are built into a meal rather than eat them, that's fine. But be careful not to exceed the fruit and veggie guidelines. As I pointed out in chapter 3, I've categorized fruit as an energy accessory because this food group typically provides about four times as much carbohydrate per serving as veggies. Also, some veggies are higher in starch and lower in water than most, which is why I created a starchy vegetable category among the energy accessory options (see page 78). When you consume fruits and starchy veggies like beets and carrots in juice form, they go down in a few gulps. Because you're not chewing them, and juice takes up less space in your stomach than fruit, it's easy to consume a higher dose of carbohydrate without feeling as full as you would if you consumed the same amount whole. Also, juice can have little fiber, depending on how the juice is made.

Yes, juicing can help you fit in more fruits and veggies, and about 75 percent of Americans fall short of the minimum recommended five daily servings. But juicing can also lead to getting too much of a good thing. The vitamins, minerals, and antioxidants in juice don't contain any calories, but juices can pack surplus carbs that either prevent weight loss or lead to weight gain. (For a more detailed explanation, see page 80.) Bottom line: Think about how the fruits and veggies you're considering juicing fit into the plan, and then adjust if needed. For example, you may decide to cook a starchy vegetable like carrots as an energy accessory rather than juice it. And if all of the veggies you're juicing are included in the vegetable list on page 73, remember that each meal should include one to two servings of veggies—1 to 2 cups raw, before going into the juicer—or 4 to 8 ounces of 100 percent vegetable juice.

Do I have to eat all of the foods in a meal at the same time?

Aim to eat the three diet wardrobe staples (lean protein, veggies, and plant-based fat) at the same time. Eating this trio together will leave you feeling more satisfied than eating each staple at a separate time, and your stomach will empty at a slower rate so you'll stay fuller longer. Eating the energy accessory with the trio can help better regulate your blood sugar and insulin levels, so this is what I recommend. But sometimes I do like to leave my energy accessory out of a meal so I can enjoy it before or after. This strategy can come in handy in several situations. For example, if you're going out to dinner, you might opt to eat a serving of grapes before you head to the restaurant, so you won't get too hungry and fall prey to the bread basket. Or if you'd like to enjoy popcorn while you watch your favorite TV show, you can save it for the after-dinner hours. There are only two rules of thumb you shouldn't break:

1. Don't move an energy accessory from one meal to another. In other words, don't eat an extra serving of whole grain, starchy vegetable, fruit, or pulse at lunch and omit it at dinner.
2. If you choose not to eat the energy accessory with the three diet wardrobe staples, be sure to eat it within three hours. So if you eat dinner at 6 P.M., enjoy that popcorn no later than 9 P.M.

Should I feel hungry while following this plan?

You don't need to experience constant hunger in order to lose weight; in fact, you shouldn't. But within a week of establishing regularly timed meals, you should feel mild to moderate hunger at your scheduled eating times. In other words, each meal should leave you feeling full and energized for three to five hours, and then your hunger should return, a signal that it's time to refuel. This pattern of hunger is normal, and it's a sign you're in balance. In other words, you're no longer overeating, and thus feeding surplus pounds you want to shed, but neither are you undereating, and starving the lean tissue you need to nourish. If you're never hungry, you may be eating too much, or you could be out of touch with your hunger and fullness signals. In either case, it can be difficult to know if you're feeding your body more than it needs to get to and maintain your ideal weight. And if you're always hungry, you're not eating enough. This could trigger a loss of muscle and a metabolism slowdown, and as a result, compromise your weight loss. If you're having a hard time differentiating between body hunger (physical) and mind hunger (emotional), see page 289.

I work out first thing in the morning, and I don't like to eat before exercising. Can I eat after?

I don't recommend exercising on an empty stomach. You may end up breaking down muscle mass to produce energy to fuel your workout. Instead, split up your breakfast by eating the energy accessory before exercising and enjoying the three diet wardrobe staples after. Remember, your energy accessory options include a serving of whole grain, starchy vegetable, fruit, or pulse, or half servings of two of these. Good preexercise energy accessory options include ¼ cup of dry oats cooked with water (whole grain); ½ cup of cubed oven-roasted, skin-on red potatoes (starchy vegetable); 1 mini banana (fruit); or ½ cup of lentils (pulse). Afterward, chose any of the meals from chapter 5, minus the energy accessory. Or choose your own combination of lean protein, veggies, and plant-based fat from the lists in chapter 3—for example, an omelet made with 1 whole organic egg and 3 whites, with 1 to 2 cups of your favorite veggies and ¼ of a ripe avocado. This "split" will help fuel your workout, prevent the loss of precious muscle, and support postexercise recovery.

Can I omit the grains from this plan?

As I explain on page 63, I don't want you to omit the energy accessories altogether. But sometimes people ask if it's okay to omit whole grains from the energy accessory options. In my opinion, you will benefit from leaving them in, even if you follow this plan gluten free. Whole grains like wild rice, oats, and quinoa provide important B vitamins and minerals, such as zinc, copper, manganese, magnesium, phosphorus, and selenium. They also supply additional antioxidants, which are tied to weight control. And statistically, people who include whole grains in a healthy diet have lower rates of obesity, diabetes, heart disease, and certain cancers. If you're concerned that grains will prevent you from losing weight, remember that the portion limits in this plan prevent carb overload. It's eating *too many* carbs, not simply eating carbs, that causes people to go wrong with whole grains. Whole grains are not inherently fattening. In fact, I've seen people lose 100 pounds while including a serving of whole grain at every single meal. So even if you want or need to omit those grains that contain gluten, I hope you won't toss out the whole-grain category completely. Otherwise, you may miss out on the nutrients they provide as well as the texture and flavors that can add a lot of enjoyment to your meals.

Should I be worried about the sugar in this plan?

Not at all, because not all sugars are created equal. None of the current health organizations or guidelines limit sugar from whole fruits and veggies and other whole, unprocessed foods. The strictest guidelines on sugar come from the American Heart Association (AHA), and they only focus on added sugars, which include refined or concentrated sugars, like the sugar you add to your morning coffee or the sugar added by manufacturers to sweetened yogurts, cereals, and baked goods. According to the AHA, the daily target for added sugar should be no more than the equivalent of about 6 level teaspoons for women and 9 for men—that's for food and beverages combined. Because my plan includes fresh, natural foods and unsweetened beverages (other than the allowance for 1 packet of raw sugar in your morning coffee and the 1 teaspoon of blackstrap molasses in the optional Sweet and Spicy Brew), you'll automatically be limiting your intake of added sugar. And the splurges built into this plan in chapter 6 easily fall within the AHA guidelines.

Naturally occurring sugar—the type added to foods by Mother Nature, like the sugar in fruit or carrots—isn't included in the AHA limits, because it's bundled with important nutrients, including vitamins, minerals, antioxidants, fiber, and water. It's also far less concentrated. For example, 1 cup of sliced fresh strawberries contains 8 grams of naturally occurring sugar, compared to 12 grams in just 1 level tablespoon of strawberry jelly made with high-fructose corn syrup, an added sugar. As with grains, people get into trouble with sugar when they consume too much. Because the foods you'll be eating in this plan that contain naturally occurring sugar are filling and portion controlled, you won't be consuming a surplus. You can still enjoy juicy pineapple and roasted carrots while shedding pounds and inches.

Can I use natural sweeteners like stevia in this plan?

I recommend avoiding all sweeteners, even natural ones. In my experience, breaking the habit of using intense sweeteners of any kind can curb a sweet tooth, improve appetite regulation, and lead to better results. If you're used to sweetening your coffee, tea, oatmeal, or smoothies and you go cold turkey, your taste buds will adjust pretty quickly.

What about protein powders other than pea protein, like hemp and whey—how do they fit in?

Nonpulse plant-based proteins, like hemp or brown-rice protein, or a USDA-certified organic grass-fed whey protein powder, are fine to use as a lean protein source. If you incorporate these into a smoothie, choose varieties made without added sugar or any sort of sweetener. Typically a serving is 1 scoop, or about ¼ cup, which can provide as much protein as a 3-ounce skinless chicken breast.

Why doesn't your plan include tofu or edamame? Has your stance on soy changed?

Yes, as a result of my personal experience. Before I started writing this book, I began struggling with intense fatigue. I'm normally full of energy, so when I found standing up in the shower to be taxing, I knew something was wrong. In addition to constantly feeling tired, I also experienced other troublesome symptoms, including brain fog, headaches, severe eczema, and extreme bloating. When going gluten free didn't make my symptoms disappear, I scheduled an appointment with my internist. After several tests found nothing wrong, my husband suggested eliminating soy. I had been eating one to two servings of soy daily, but they were always USDA-certified organic, whole soy foods, which I enjoyed and had always believed to be healthful. But I was desperate for relief, so I took my hubby's suggestion and avoided all soy.

Within a week, I started to feel better. After a few weeks, my energy was returning, and I began to feel like myself again. Then something happened that convinced me that I indeed had a problem with soy. I accidently consumed soy in a sauce, and almost instantly I felt like my belly was on fire. I was itchy, my head throbbed, and within fifteen minutes I looked four months pregnant (I have photos to document my "soy belly"). Jack was right: soy seemed to be triggering my symptoms. As I talked to colleagues about my experience, nearly everyone had a comparable story to share about a client, patient, or family member.

I believe that, as we've seen with the surge in gluten intolerance, we may see a rise in soy intolerance, which appears to have a similar set of symptoms. (For more about gluten intolerance, see page 275.) In any case, because I've had to say good-bye to soy, I chose not to include it as a lean protein option in this plan. But if you don't experience any problems with soy, just as some don't with gluten, and you'd like to include it in your diet, I encourage you to consume only USDA-certified organic, whole soy foods. The following amounts comprise one serving:

- one-fifth of a 14-ounce package of extra-firm tofu
- ½ cup of edamame
- 1 cup (8 ounces) of whole soy milk

I also encourage you to monitor your body's reactions, because, as I found, your body may begin to rebel at any time.

Can I drink alcohol?

I think the answer depends on your relationship with alcohol. Over the years, many of my clients have told me that having one drink on the weekend turned into imbibing two or three or more, which led to some serious overeating. As a result, they canceled out a week's worth of healthy eating and remained stuck on a weight-loss plateau. One recent survey found that in a single evening, 40 percent of women consume on average

1,000 calories in alcoholic drinks alone. And four in five reported that drinking diminishes their willpower, causing them to indulge in foods like burgers, pizza, and chips. If alcohol tends to be your diet downfall, consider becoming a teetotaler for at least thirty days, or until you've lost a significant amount of weight. When you do feel comfortable adding alcohol back into your diet, use the strategies I've laid out starting on page 283 to prevent one drink from snowballing into a serious binge.

Can I season my meals with sea salt?

If you do not have high blood pressure, you can sprinkle a small amount of sea salt or a specialty salt, like pink Himalayan or *fleur de sel,* on your oven-roasted red potatoes or baked salmon. But keep in mind that the recommended daily intake for sodium is 1,500 to 2,300 milligrams per day. This total includes the sodium naturally found in whole, fresh foods (for example, 1 cup of chopped raw carrots contains 88 milligrams of sodium), the sodium added to processed foods like bread, and the sodium in salt (which is made from a combination of 40 percent sodium and 60 percent chloride). Aim for the lower limit—1,500 milligrams—if you're fifty-one or older, or African American, or if you have high blood pressure, diabetes, or chronic kidney disease.

Americans typically get about 70 percent of their sodium intake from processed foods, like frozen dinners, canned soups, and snack foods. Because my plan is based primarily on fresh, unprocessed foods, you'll automatically be slashing your sodium intake. But some choices within the plan—like canned pulses, whole-grain crackers, and whole-grain bread—may cause your sodium intake to creep up. Because even fresh vegetables provide some sodium, and I know you'll consume more from certain packaged foods, I have opted not to use salt as a seasoning in my recipes.

When I tested the recipes in chapter 5, I was very pleased with their flavors, and they passed my hubby's taste test without added salt. However, if you're concerned that you may not be getting enough sodium, particularly if you lose sodium by sweating during exercise, you may want to add a small amount after cooking. Just keep in mind that 1 level teaspoon of sea salt contains over 2,300 milligrams of sodium, a full day's worth or more, depending on your personal needs. So, we're talking about scant amounts, such as ¹⁄₁₆ teaspoon, which provides less than 150 milligrams of sodium. Just this tiny amount is plenty for adding flavor to roasted Brussels sprouts or Oven-Roasted Sweet Potato "Fries."

As for the benefits of sea salt, which is made from evaporated seawater, it's certainly more natural than table salt, which is typically mined from underground salt deposits, processed to eliminate minerals, and treated with anticlumping agents. Sea salt also retains traces of minerals, such as magnesium, potassium, and calcium. Though the amounts of these nutrients aren't significant, their presence does add flavor, which is why you won't need to use more than a tiny pinch. If you think you may be using too much, measure out ¹⁄₁₆ teaspoon (it's more than you might think!), place it in a ramekin, and keep track of how much you're using, rather than sprinkling it straight from a shaker.

I've been hearing a lot about sprouted grains. Are they included in this plan?

Sprouted grains, like sprouted whole wheat, sprouted brown rice, and sprouted rye, have become popular in recent years. Essentially, grain kernels contain the raw materials needed to grow a new plant, so when the temperature and moisture conditions are just right, the kernel will sprout into a new baby plant. Part of the process involves enzymes, which trigger the grain to sprout. These same enzymes allow the baby plant to digest the starch in the kernel, which supplies its fuel, and boost the accessibility of nutrients, to promote the plant's growth. Fans of sprouted grains say that when we eat these plants, we enjoy these same benefits—easier to digest starch and more nutrients. Sprouted grains may also be slightly higher in protein than other types of grains, because some carbohydrates are lost in the process of sprouting. And you still get the benefits of eating a whole grain.

Consuming some sprouted grains can be a nice way to broaden the spectrum of your healthy diet. However, at this time, there is no regulated definition of the term *sprouted grain,* and fresh sprouts (usually found in the produce section) are highly perishable, so it's important to check the expiration date and store them safely to prevent foodborne illness. Also, while sprouting may be beneficial, there are numerous studies to support the benefits of consuming regular (technically called *nongerminated*) whole grains, so I definitely recommend keeping them in your food repertoire.

All the diet plans I tried in the past involved counting, whether it was calories, points, or grams. Is it really possible to get results without counting?

Yes! As long as you're consistent with the portions I recommend—for example, using a level ½ cup of potatoes rather than a heaping scoop—you can enjoy terrific and lasting results without counting anything. As you can see from the success stories scattered throughout the book, the results are impressive, and these women counted nothing. And the women who previously had followed counting-based diets were happy to be free from the burden of tracking calories, grams, or points. My guess is you'll feel equally liberated.

Is this plan truly vegan friendly?

Yes. The Rapid Pulse is completely vegan, as are all of the dessert recipes in chapter 6, and the Daily Pulse can be followed with no animal foods at all. One of my favorite aspects of the plan is that it is customizable to anyone's needs and preferences. There are plenty of vegan meals in chapter 5, and in chapter 3, you'll find a do-it-yourself meal building strategy that you can easily use if you are vegan. Also, many of the meals in chapter 5 that contain dairy, eggs, poultry, or seafood as the lean protein can be made with pulses while keeping the other ingredients the same, which would make these recipes vegan. For example, cannellini beans are an excellent substitute for chicken in the cacciatore dish or for shrimp in the scampi recipe. And as you'll see from looking through the pulse recipes, mashed chickpeas work well in place of eggs in a scramble, and mashed or chopped beans can replace cheese in dishes like the Chilled Italian Stuffed Tomatoes.

If I'm making a recipe for my family of four, should I just quadruple the ingredients?

Yes. And leaving out the energy accessory or making it separately will allow you to prepare greater quantities, if needed. For example, if your hubby or kids aren't trying to lose weight, they may be able to eat a larger portion of Oven-Roasted Sweet Potato "Fries" or brown rice pasta than you can, so you may want to more than quadruple this part of the meal. However, the portions of the diet wardrobe staples should be appropriate for nearly anyone in the family. Still, for an active teenage boy or a very active man, you may need to double the portion of lean protein.

Grocery Shopping Questions

I don't have time to soak and boil dry beans. Are canned pulses okay?

Yes, but look for canned options marked "BPA free." Bisphenol A is a building block of plastics used in many packaged products, including canned foods. This chemical has been tied to a disruption in thyroid function and a greater risk of obesity. Researchers say BPA may act like estrogen in the body, and animal research has found that it accelerates the formation of fat cells. Mice exposed to BPA before birth have a greater risk of obesity, and female mice that consumed a low dose of BPA in their drinking water packed on 13 percent more body weight than mice not exposed to BPA.

Even if you can't find BPA-free cans, I still consider pulses a must-eat food. But fortunately more and more manufacturers are eliminating this chemical from packaging. Other shortcut pulse options include vacuum-sealed and frozen products. Nearly every week I buy vacuum-sealed steamed lentils in the produce section of my market. I also regularly buy frozen bags of precooked black-eyed peas, chickpeas, and lentils. The vacuum-sealed lentils can be eaten chilled or warmed up, and the frozen pulses can be thawed in the fridge and eaten chilled or heated from frozen. If you're sodium conscious, frozen options are a terrific choice. A ½ cup serving of frozen pulse contains less than 10 milligrams of sodium, compared to nearly 250 milligrams in the vacuum-sealed bag and 450 milligrams in a canned product. When you do opt for canned, look for products labeled "no added salt," which can reduce the sodium to as little as 10 milligrams per ½ cup. If you can't find no-added-salt cans, rinsing helps. Washing pulses in a colander under the faucet can remove about 40 percent of the sodium in any canned product.

What are heirloom beans?

There is no standard definition of *heirloom,* but the term usually refers to seeds that have been passed down from generation to generation. Other definitions describe heirlooms as plants that are grown traditionally on a small scale, using seeds from varieties that are at least fifty years old, but some heirloom plants are much older. In short, farmers and growers save the seeds from their best plants, including those that are the most hearty (which can mean more nutritious), flavorful, and beautiful. Many heirlooms have unusual shapes and colors, which differentiate them from commercial plants, which are typically bred to produce uniform-looking, high-yielding, inexpensive crops. For these reasons, heirlooms are generally pricier. You can find heirloom beans in the bulk section of many health food stores, but a branded 12-ounce bag of dry heirloom beans may cost $5 to $6, compared to roughly $2 to $3 for a 16-ounce bag of common beans. You might opt to use heirloom beans for special-occasion meals or those where the beans are visually the centerpieces of a dish. Some of my favorite varieties include

- Appaloosa
- Black Calypso
- Black Valentine

- Christmas Lima
- Rio Zape
- Scarlet Runner
- Sunset Runner

If you Google these delicious gems, you'll find images of their gorgeous shapes and colors as well as information about where to purchase or order them. Also, be sure to check your local farmers' market. The first time I saw Christmas Lima beans was at the Union Square Greenmarket in New York City. If you visit www.sustainabletable.org, you can find your local farmers' markets as well as shops in your area that sell local, organic, and artisan goods.

Can I use store-bought hummus?

Yes, just read the full ingredient list to be sure that it's all natural. Also, most premade varieties of hummus include olive oil, tahini, or both, which means that the plant-based fat is included. And I bet you'll like this: You can eat twice as much as 2 tablespoons, the serving stated on the label. That's because 4 tablespoons, or ¼ cup, is closer to the amount you'd get if you made the hummus yourself, starting with ½ cup of chickpeas. When you do have time for homemade, you'll enjoy even more volume, as well as more filling protein and fiber, than commercial varieties provide. If you've never made it yourself, give it a try. You'll find a traditional chickpea-based recipe in chapter 5, flavored with garlic, lemon, and black pepper, as well as a version made with black beans, seasoned with cilantro and pureed with ripe avocado.

Is it okay to buy flavored yogurt?

Yes, as long as it's USDA-certified organic and nonfat. Plain, unsweetened, fat-free Greek yogurt contains 6 grams of naturally occurring sugar in a single-serving container. The same-size portion of vanilla yogurt contains 12 grams. That means roughly 6 grams of sugar, about 1½ teaspoons, are added, since every 4 grams of added sugar equals a teaspoon. That's still very little compared to the added-sugar limits advised by the American Heart Association (see page 264). So if you really can't stand the sourness of plain, a sweetened variety is fine. In fact, when I was testing the recipes in chapter 5, I found that some, like the Lemon Mint Avocado Smoothie, just didn't work with plain yogurt, but it came out great with vanilla. So that single teaspoon and a half of added sugar can make a big difference, without adding much sugar to your overall daily intake.

What if I can't find nonfat organic cottage and ricotta cheeses?

If you can't find a brand that's both fat free and USDA-certified organic, look for one that's either fat free and all natural (no hormones or antibiotics, no artificial additives) or reduced-fat organic.

How can I avoid GMOs?

GMO stands for "genetically modified organism." Genetic modification allows DNA from one species to be injected into another species to create combinations of plant, animal, bacteria, and viral genes that don't occur in nature or through traditional crossbreeding methods. Though the unintended effects of genetic engineering are unclear, many experts are concerned about the potential for possible allergic reactions and hidden illnesses as well as superpests and superweeds (bugs and weeds that become resistant to chemicals that have been used to keep them under control).

In Europe, food products that contain more than 0.9 percent GMO are required by the government to be labeled. In the United States, consumers aren't able to tell which foods contain GMOs, and it's estimated that they may be present in more than 75 percent of the processed foods in your average grocery store. Right now, one of the best ways to avoid them is to look for USDA-certified organic foods, which can't be grown using GM ingredients. However, that's not practical 100 percent of the time. And while GMO seeds and ingredients are not supposed to be used in organic products, no testing is required to show whether cross-pollination or contamination has occurred. For this reason, it's also helpful to look for products that carry the Non-GMO Project Verified seal, which indicates that a product has been tested for GM ingredients. You can also use their free app to search by product type, brand name, product name, and key word.

I heard that the additive carrageenan in foods like almond and coconut milk is unhealthy. Should I try to avoid it?

Yes. Carrageenan is a natural food additive derived from seaweed that is used as a thickener and stabilizer. One researcher who has studied carrageenan extensively, Joanne K. Tobacman at the University of Illinois College of Medicine, believes it causes inflammation, a known trigger of premature aging and diseases, including obesity. What's more, one of Dr. Tobacman's animal studies found that this additive interfered with blood sugar and insulin regulation, and may therefore increase the risk of type 2 diabetes. Fortunately, you can find products free from carrageenan, and more and more companies are removing it. However, brands are constantly reformulating, so always read ingredient lists.

Personal Health Questions

Can I follow this plan gluten free?

Yes. Three of the energy accessory options—starchy vegetables, fruit, and pulses—are naturally gluten-free starches. You can also select gluten-free whole-grain options from the lists in chapter 3, including buckwheat soba noodles, corn, quinoa, and wild and brown rice. For packaged items and grain products that traditionally contain gluten, like whole-grain crackers and bread, you can certainly use gluten-free versions—whole-grain brown rice pasta, for example, is one of my favorites.

Is a gluten-free diet healthier?

For some people, yes, but for others, I think the jury is still out. You've now read my personal saga with soy. Many of my clients have experienced a very similar struggle with gluten and feel significantly better once they've removed it from their diets. Others feel absolutely fine when they eat 100 percent whole-grain bread or other whole, unprocessed grains that naturally contain gluten, such as barley, particularly USDA-certified organic versions of these foods.

What exactly is gluten, and why is it harmful for some people? Gluten is a type of protein naturally found in wheat (including spelt, kamut, farro, and bulgur) and other grains, like barley and rye. In people who have celiac disease, consuming even a tiny amount of gluten triggers severe abdominal pain, bloating, and other debilitating symptoms. This happens because gluten causes the immune system to damage or destroy villi, the tiny, fingerlike outgrowths that line the small intestine and help absorb nutrients through the intestinal wall into the bloodstream. Damaged villi cause chronic malnutrition, typically accompanied by exhaustion and weight loss. Other symptoms of celiac disease include bone or joint pain, depression, and skin problems. In people diagnosed with celiac, the only way to reverse the damage and eliminate the symptoms is to completely avoid gluten. But many people who test negative for celiac disease nonetheless experience troubling side effects from consuming gluten. These people suffer from a condition called *gluten intolerance* or *gluten sensitivity*. Though not as serious as celiac disease, gluten intolerance can cause flu-like feelings, bloating and other gastrointestinal problems, mental fogginess, and fatigue. Unfortunately, there is no accurate test for gluten sensitivity at this time (hopefully there's one on the way), but avoiding gluten tends to relieve the symptoms.

If you're not sure whether you're sensitive to gluten, you might try eliminating gluten for a week, or even a full month, and monitoring your energy level, mood, and digestive health. If you're confident that you feel just fine after consuming foods with gluten, I don't think you need to avoid it, especially in this plan. That's because you'll be eating all-natural, whole-grain versions of foods that naturally contain gluten, rather than processed foods that have been stripped of their nutrients and loaded up with artificial additives. In my experience, one of the reasons people feel so great and lose weight when they ditch gluten is because they go from eating terribly unhealthy, carb-dense processed foods, like cookies, crackers, white bagels, and pasta, to eating more veggies and high-fiber, nutrient-rich foods, like produce, pulses, and quinoa.

I heard it's important to start the day with warm lemon water. Is this true?

Drinking warm lemon water first thing in the morning is an Ayurvedic practice. (Ayurveda is a form of alternative medicine native to India.) The philosophy is that the combination of lemon and water hydrates, helps with digestion (because warm water stimulates the muscles of the GI tract), balances pH (while lemon seems acidic, it's alkaline in terms of how it's metabolized), supports immunity (due to the lemon's vitamin C), and helps with weight loss. The latter may be true—higher blood levels of vitamin C have been tied in research to increased fat burning, and hydration is important for optimal metabolism. Though I don't tell all of my clients that drinking lemon water is something they must do every day, it definitely has benefits. So if you'd like to adopt this ritual, go for it.

Since I started following the plan, people tell me my skin looks better. Could this possibly be due to my new eating habits?

Absolutely. Hands down, fruits and veggies are the most important ingredients for healthy, glowing skin, and you're eating plenty of both as part of this plan. In one study, scientists tracked the diets of thirty-five adults, took photos of them, and asked others to rate the pictures. The volunteers who consumed an average of 2.9 more portions of fruits and vegetables each day were rated as healthier looking, and those who consumed an extra 3.3 portions daily were rated as more attractive. A similar study in the United Kingdom found that pictures of volunteers who ate a fruit- and veggie-rich diet were rated as more attractive than those with suntans. The reason? Antioxidants. Scientists say they alter skin pigment and improve circulation, increasing blood flow to the skin's surface. Antioxidants also act like natural bodyguards against skin-damaging toxins, including cigarette smoke, pollution, and internal substances produced as a result of stress and sun exposure. So every time you make a meal in this plan, you're literally eating your way to better looks!

Will this eating plan help my hair look healthier?

Yes. When you are well hydrated and maintain good circulation, two benefits of this plan, you'll have a much healthier scalp, which can have a big impact on how your hair lies on your head and how thick it appears. Also, each time you lose a hair (you lose, on average, 50 to 150 strands per day), a new hair sprouts from the same follicle, and its quality is largely based on your diet. The nutrient-rich foods in this plan and the balance provided by the combination of lean protein, veggies, plant-based fats, and healthy energy accessories can help optimize the maintenance, repair, and regeneration of every cell in your body, from head to toe.

Can I follow this plan while pregnant, not for weight loss but just as a healthy way of eating?

Not as the plan is presented. While my plan is very healthy, I didn't design it with the needs of a pregnant woman in mind. A modified version may be fine, but please get your doctor's approval and guidance. You might even bring your doctor the book and ask how you should adjust the plan to meet your pregnancy needs. For example, he or she may recommend four daily meals, at least two full servings of energy accessories at each meal, and possibly more protein. Only your physician can provide you with this kind of individualized advice.

Can I follow this plan while breastfeeding?

I did not create the plan with breastfeeding needs in mind. My general advice would be that a breastfeeding mom should definitely skip the Rapid Pulse. Also, she should include two full servings of energy accessories at

each meal and possibly add a fourth meal. But as I stated in the front of
this book, always consult your doctor about the best eating plan for your
personal needs.

How can I quit using artificial sweeteners?

I'm so glad that you're ready to stop using artificial sweeteners. Recent
research supports what I've seen in my private practice for years: artificial sweeteners may actually increase sweet cravings. Scientists say this is
because fake sugars activate the brain's pleasure center without satisfying it,
triggering an increased desire for sweets. That's probably why, statistically,
people who drink diet beverages aren't slimmer; in fact, people who drink
diet soda are statistically more likely to be overweight or obese than those
who drink regular soda. Of course, I'm not advocating drinking regular
soda, but if you're worried that giving up faux sugars will lead to weight
gain, I'm confident you'll find the opposite result.

After kicking the diet soda habit, my clients always report fewer cravings for sweets, a heightened ability to tune in to hunger and fullness
cues, and far more effortless weight loss. I think the best approach may
be to go cold turkey, then start a cravings journal. In addition to tracking what and how much you eat, record your hunger and fullness ratings
before and after meals (see page 289) as well as any observations related
to cravings. If you're still experiencing cravings, choose fresh, sweet, juicy
fruit as your energy accessory (or a half serving along with a half serving
of another option) to satisfy your sweet tooth. You might also try using
"sweet" spices. Though not technically sweet themselves, spices such as
ginger, cinnamon, clove, cardamom, and nutmeg enhance natural sweetness. You can sprinkle them into your morning cup of coffee or onto a
baked sweet potato, or stir them into oatmeal, natural nut butter, or nonfat organic Greek yogurt. Finally, you can enjoy some real sugar without
blowing your weight-loss results. Check out the decadent pulse dessert
recipes in chapter 6, and see page 301 for savvy ways to build in other
can't-live-without splurges. In my experience, avoiding artificial sweeten-

ers and indulging in small amounts of the real thing is the best way to satisfy your fix and move on.

I have been hearing a lot about the importance of an alkaline diet. Is this plan alkaline friendly?

Yes. Diets aimed at reducing metabolic acidity are becoming increasingly popular, and some recent research has found merit in this eating strategy. When the foods you eat are metabolized, compounds are generated that either promote acidity or form alkaline substances, which neutralize acidity. Generally, animal proteins are particularly acid forming, whereas fruits and vegetables are alkalizing.

One study, which tracked over sixty-five thousand women for fourteen years, found that a high acid load can interfere with proper insulin function. In the study, eating in a way that increased acidity was tied to a 56 percent greater risk of developing type 2 diabetes. This study is in line with dozens of others that demonstrate the benefits of reducing animal proteins and eating more plant-based meals. Even if you aren't interested in becoming a vegetarian, this plan will help you shift to a more plant-based way of eating.

One challenge with alkaline diets is that you can't tell, intuitively, which foods are alkaline and which are acidic. For example, lemons and apple cider vinegar, which both seem acidic, are considered alkaline because of how they are metabolized in the body. Also, the acid-forming list includes some very healthy foods, such as cranberries, pomegranates, and walnuts. Additionally, in searching online, I found conflicting versions of the alkaline/acidic charts. Some foods, like quinoa, appear on an alkaline list in one chart but an acidic list in another. In my opinion, you don't need to memorize or refer to complicated lists, because the best way to improve your acid-to-alkaline balance is to simply eat fewer animal foods and more plants. And the way my plan is designed, even if you include one serving of animal protein at every meal, only three of the roughly twelve to twenty foods you'll be eating each day will be animal foods, and many of the foods you'll enjoy will be highly alkaline. So even if some of the plant foods you choose metabolize to acid, you'll likely still fall within the minimum 60 percent alkaline range most proponents recommend.

I've noticed that since I began following this plan, I just feel happier.
Can that be?

You bet. Far and away the most potent foods for improving mood are fruits and vegetables, and you're eating plenty of them in this plan. One study, published in the *British Journal of Health Psychology,* asked young adults to complete daily food diaries, including psychological and mood-related ratings, for three consecutive weeks. Compared to the volunteers who ate low amounts of produce, those who piled on the fruits and veggies reported having more energy and feeling calmer and happier, not just on the days they ate lots of produce but also on the days following. Another study, published in the journal *Social Indicators Research,* tracked the eating habits of eighty thousand adults and found that consuming more fruits and veggies enhanced mental well-being. The magic number for happiness was seven servings a day. Since you'll be eating one to two portions of veggies in each of your three daily meals, and you can choose fruit or starchy vegetables as your energy accessories, you can easily hit that mark day after day.

[10]

Day 31 and Beyond

Congratulations on completing the 30-day challenge! In the last four weeks, you've revved up your metabolism, nourished yourself with healthy cuisine, and learned a whole new meal-building strategy that allows you to lose weight while optimizing your health and well-being. You've also adopted a powerful daily meditation practice and transformed your relationship with food, physical activity, and your body. These are huge accomplishments, so I think you owe yourself a big pat on the back—even an unabashed "I did it!"

By this time, I hope that the meals, techniques, and information in this book have dispelled the notion that your old, restrictive "diet" approaches to weight loss are the only ones that work, and that the healthy habits you've established have begun to feel like your new normal. If you haven't yet reached your weight goal, continue with my plan and you'll keep making progress. And if you have hit your target (woo-hoo!), I hope you will adopt this plan as a way of life, to maintain your results and continue to maximize your energy and health. Unlike thirty-day "diets" that require deprivation and aren't sustainable over the long haul, my plan—as I hope you've discovered!—is one you can maintain. After all, it does include can't-live-without splurges.

Still, I want to acknowledge that obstacles are bound to surface now and again. A vacation, a holiday party, a happy-hour gathering with coworkers, a particularly busy or emotional week—these all have the potential to throw you off. So, to stick with the plan, you may need some new skills. In this chapter I share strategies for preventing and/or overcoming the ten most common challenges my clients encounter, so that a minor hiccup doesn't jolt you off track. I also show you how to build in splurges in a way that allows you to maintain your results. You've worked hard and ventured a long way. I want to help keep you on the healthy path you have forged.

Social Snacking

I mentioned that now and then I leave the energy accessory out of my meal so I can save it for later. This strategy allows me to munch on popcorn while I watch my favorite TV show, which I sometimes do because it's difficult to watch my hubby snack beside me. At times, a mug of tea or glass of water just doesn't cut it. As long as you've planned your snack in advance and have prepared an amount that fits into this plan, snacking while watching the boob tube can actually be a smart tactic, because it fits with your social life. The same may be true of snacking at other times of day. Let's say you enjoy an afternoon snack with a coworker. If your My Energy Needs quiz on page 87 indicates that you don't need a snack in addition to your three daily meals, you can save the energy accessory, or even half of it, like ½ cup of fresh grapes, to enjoy at this time. As I noted on page 262, the only rule of thumb is to eat this portion of your meal within three hours. So if you have lunch at noon, aim for a midafternoon energy accessory snack no later than 3 P.M.

If you find yourself snacking out of habit rather than hunger (for example, you always have nuts as soon as you get home), make an effort to change up your routine. If you tend to turn on the TV and snack while you sort through your mail, turn on music instead, save the mail for later, and immediately start prepping for dinner. Sometimes just altering a pattern can break a bad habit. When you disconnect eating from specific activities, your brain can begin to let go of the notion that it doesn't feel "right" not to do these things simultaneously. Your new routines may seem forced or awkward at first, but before long, the healthier patterns will feel natural and normal.

Dealing with Alcohol

This is a biggie. Few of my clients are interested in giving up alcohol completely, but many know that imbibing often triggers overeating. And alcoholic beverages themselves can pack a ton of surplus carbohydrates. For example, one 12-ounce regular beer typically contains as much carbohydrate as a slice of bread. Just 4 ounces (½ cup) of a sweetened mixer clocks in at 25 grams of carbs, about fourteen gummy bears' worth. If becoming a teetotaler doesn't feel right for you, you can still enjoy a cocktail now and then without undoing your healthy efforts. Here's how:

Eat before you take your first sip.

When your stomach is empty, alcohol is absorbed quickly, which means you'll feel the effects within minutes.

*Know the definition of **moderation**.*

Technically, 12 ounces of light beer (one bottle or can), 5 ounces of wine (a little smaller than a yogurt container), and 1.5 ounces (1 shot) of liquor all pack about the same amount of alcohol, so each is considered one standard drink. The guidelines for moderation advise no more than one standard drink per day for women, two for men. And no, they don't carry over to the next day. In other words you can't have none all week and seven drinks on Saturday! If you're not sure whether you're overdoing it, track your alcohol intake for a week or two. Many of my clients who perceived themselves as light drinkers have discovered by logging that they drink far more than moderately (see page 290).

If you're a beer drinker, choose a low-carb option.

A 12-ounce bottle or can of ultra-low-carb beer contains about 3 to 4 grams of carbs, compared to at least 10 grams—about as much as 10 mini pretzels—in a regular version.

Mind your mixers.

If you drink liquor, become discriminating about what it's mixed with. Just 4 ounces of cola contains about 12 grams of carbohydrate, and the same amount of sour mix will cost you a whopping 25 grams of carbs. A smart strategy is to ask for soda water or club soda with lemon or lime as your mixer; unlike tonic, soda water and club soda are naturally carb free. At home, add an antioxidant boost by tossing in muddled fresh fruit, like berries, and an herb, such as fresh grated ginger or mint leaves.

Slow down, and sip water.

Getting too tipsy too fast is one of the biggest culprits in alcohol-induced overeating. To temper the rise of your blood alcohol level, order a tall glass of water with every alcoholic beverage. Alternate sips, and finish at least 12 ounces of water for every cocktail.

Avoid mindlessly munching.

If you're at a bar with free happy-hour munchies, like popcorn or nuts, turn your back on them or place them out of arm's reach. When food is directly in front of you, you're likely to grab it without even realizing it, even if you aren't hungry. The odds definitely increase after a cocktail or two.

Plan your postdrinking meal.

Scope out nearby restaurants in advance, so you can suggest a spot that accommodates this plan.

YOU MAY BE DRINKING MORE THAN YOU THINK

Restaurant servings of wine and liquor are about 40 percent larger than the amounts considered to be standard, according to one recent study. Another report found that the alcohol levels in beer and wine are increasing, so you may be getting up to 50 percent more alcohol than you think. Also, if you order beer by the pint (16 ounces), you'll take in 4 ounces above the standard drink amount, and if your bartender doesn't use a shot glass to measure liquor, you could easily be consuming much more than 1.5 ounces. So pay attention to the alcohol you order and how it's served. Otherwise, you could become tipsier than you bargained for. The resulting combination of an appetite spike and lowered inhibitions could prompt you to reach for foods you wouldn't choose while sober.

VOLUNTEER TO BE THE DESIGNATED DRIVER

I've had clients give up alcohol and drop weight like a hot potato. So if you're serious about weight loss, your best strategy may be to avoid drinking altogether. One smart way to do so without sacrificing your social life is to volunteer to drive. It's a great way to save your group taxi or ride-sharing costs, and while it may not be as fun as indulging with your group, you'll wake up the next day without a hangover or regrets, and that feels pretty darn good.

Weekend Indulgences

For most of my clients, the chances of veering off track are much greater on the weekends, largely because weekends are when most of us have hours of unstructured time. This deviation from the normal routine can lead to wandering into the kitchen and extra nibbling, or using food to fill time, like grabbing a vanilla latte or frozen yogurt.

If this sounds like you, add structure to your weekend days by planning a project or activity you enjoy, along with a built-in deadline. For example, start a craft project, like jewelry making, needlepoint, or mosaic art, and plan to give your creation to a friend or family member or donate it on a specific date. Once you've finished a project, start another. Adding purposeful activities to Saturdays and Sundays can keep your mind and hands busy and end what some of my clients refer to as "two-day food orgies." Taking up a new hobby can also add to your quality of life in numerous ways, giving you a creative outlet and boosting your mood.

WHY WEEKDAYS COUNT MOST

A Cornell University study that tracked 80 adults for up to 330 days found that nearly all of the subjects ate more and experienced weight fluctuations on the weekends. However, it was their weekday behavior that determined if they lost weight long term. Compared to people who gained weight, those who lost weight over the course of the study got back on track on Monday and were consistent during the week. This study doesn't mean you should throw caution to the wind every Saturday and Sunday, but it does indicate that if you do get a little off track on the weekends, your weekday choices can still allow you to lose weight.

Emotional Eating

We're socialized to use food emotionally. We bond over meals, and we use food to celebrate, show our affection, and comfort ourselves and the people we care about. After all my years counseling clients, I'm certain that overcoming emotional eating is one the most important steps you can take to shed pounds. Here are the four most effective ways to prevent your emotions from getting the best of you.

Express your feelings.

A friend's therapist once advised her to buy cheap dishes at a garage sale, take them into her backyard, and smash them to bits. She followed through—with a single dish—and she said it was one of the most liberating moments of her life. Now, I'm not a therapist, and I'm not recommending this technique (who wants to clean that up?!), but in my practice, I have seen that walking around with bottled-up emotions considerably increases the chances that you'll use food to stuff down your feelings or detach from them. So it's important to find healthy ways to release your emotions, like watching a tearjerker to have a good cry when you're sad or aggressively cleaning when you're angry.

Distance yourself from trigger foods.

Numerous clients have told me they can't keep certain foods around, because if the foods are there, they'll eat them, especially when they're emotional. However, unless you live alone, it can be impossible to banish high-risk foods completely. The solution is to make trigger foods harder to access. Studies show that the fewer steps you have to take to get to a food, the more likely you are to eat it, and vice versa. So stash candy or cookies on a higher shelf, wrapped in another bag or inside a sealed container. Place ice cream in the back of the freezer behind bags of frozen fruits and veggies. In addition to being practical, this distance can buy you the time to consider other options. One client told me this trick make her think,

"Hmm, I can either go in the closet, get the step stool, and pull down the candy, or I can call my friend." In that moment, picking up the phone just seemed easier, and after she hung up, she no longer felt drawn to the hidden goodies.

Catch your emotions before they become too intense.

Strong emotions tend to drown out rational thoughts, distancing you from the consequences of emotional eating. In other words, when you're really sad, angry, or scared, you know that eating ice cream will make you feel better right that minute, which makes it easy to push away thoughts about your weight or how you'll feel tomorrow. When you catch your emotions before they become too forceful, you're more likely to address them in ways that don't involve food, alcohol, or both. It's not easy, and it doesn't happen overnight, but make a conscious effort to tune in to what it feels like when your emotions are building. For example, you might experience an upset stomach, tense jaw, neck or shoulder tension, or shallow breathing. When you notice these symptoms, stop, take a deep breath or meditate, and express or address what you're feeling.

If you do eat emotionally, do so with awareness.

If you find yourself reaching for chips or chocolate because you're sad or anxious, and you can't or don't want to find an alternative, eat while sitting in a chair and without distractions. Most of my clients eat emotionally while watching TV, reading, surfing the web, or listening to music. When you take away that second activity, emotion-driven eating may feel incredibly awkward, but that's a good thing. When you're preoccupied, it's easy to lose track of how fast and how much you're eating. But eating emotionally with full awareness can seem like going from being in the dark to turning the lights on. Chances are, you'll eat a lot less or realize that eating doesn't feel like the best way to cope.

••

ARE YOU HONEST WITH YOURSELF ABOUT YOUR HABITS?

We all fib a little now and again. Some little white lies are harmless, like telling your coworker her new haircut looks great (when what you're really thinking is "Oh my!"). But fibbing to yourself about the healthfulness of your own eating and activity habits isn't so innocent, because it can wreak some real emotional and physical havoc. With my private practice clients, I make it very clear from the start that my job isn't to scold or berate them, or act like a food cop. In fact, it's just the opposite. As their food counselor, I want to help them foster open, honest, nonjudgmental communication about their relationships with food. And that can't be accomplished if some truths are being pushed under the rug. Here are four untruths many of my clients eventually reveal, and when they come clean, these fibs are no longer holding them back from the weight-loss and health results that have eluded them. As you read through them, check in to see if it's time to get truthful about your own habits.

"I eat when I'm hungry and stop when I'm full."

I have many clients who claim to only eat when they feel hungry and stop when they're full. Yet when I review their food diaries, I frequently see snacks just an hour or two after fairly substantial meals, when they shouldn't yet be experiencing bodily sensations of hunger. When I ask "What did the hunger feel like?" it often turns out to be emotional or social rather than physical in nature. In other words, there were no physical symptoms that signaled a need for energy or nourishment, and in truth, the client often knows this to be true. Some will say things like "I knew I wasn't really hungry, but I didn't know what else to do with myself, so I nibbled." In other words, the desire to eat was more about anxiety or boredom than the physical need for food. One of the best ways to recognize the difference is to keep a food diary, which includes not just what you eat and how much but also your hunger level before and after meals, in addition to your emotions. Once you're able to differentiate bodily hunger (which has physical signs and symptoms, like a growling stomach) from nonphysical hunger, you can work on finding other, healthy ways to address with what's really going on (stress, relationship issues, and so on). As a result, you'll stop overfeeding yourself and start seeing a lot more weight-loss progress.

"I'm not a big drinker."

I've heard this from many clients who meet the criteria of the Centers for Disease Control and Prevention (CDC) for chronic binge drinking. The technical definition of binge drinking is the consumption of four or more drinks in a two-hour period for women, or five for men. According to the CDC, one in six adults binge drinks about four times a month. And according to a recent study from the University of Texas at Austin, even when overall alcohol intake is still moderate, sporadic binge drinking increases mortality risk. Scientists say this is because binge drinking concentrates alcohol's toxicity, which can damage organs, and increases the risk of accidents. So, if you don't drink Sunday through Thursday but you go to a happy hour Friday night and have four drinks in the two hours after work, you're not drinking "in moderation." In addition to the health risks, this pattern can also hold you back from seeing weight-loss results. Many of my clients who binge drink believe they aren't big drinkers, because they've already cut back, or because they're comparing themselves to friends who drink a lot more or more often. But after some reflection, I often hear sentiments like "I know polishing off a bottle of wine by myself isn't good, even if it's only on the weekends." If this routine sounds familiar, think about the reasons for your drinking. Perhaps you're using alcohol as an emotional crutch or it's integral to your social scene. Connecting with a close friend or family member who supports your decision to cut back can help tremendously. And in my experience, curbing alcohol intake often leads to feeling "cleaner," more in control, and more motivated to eat healthfully and be active—changes that can be transformative for both your waistline and your health.

"I eat really healthfully most of the time."

Many of my clients tell me that they "really try" to eat well, but when we actually talk about their usual meals, they include portions of starch that are way too large, too few vegetables, too much cheese and meat, and too many unplanned indulgences. No, they're not pigging out on fast food or candy or drinking sugary beverages, but they're also not consistently eating in ways that allow them to achieve and maintain a healthy weight. After acknowledging this, one of my clients admitted that she had been looking at her diet through rose-colored glasses. She said, "I think I was giving myself an A when what I really earned was more like a B– or C+." Perfection isn't the goal, but shedding some light on just how far off you are from what's optimal (for example, this plan) can allow you to set some concrete goals that will get the scale moving in the right direction, and allow you to feel better as well.

"I work out a lot."

I work with professional athletes, models, and entertainers whose performances are very physical, but most of my clients are women and men who work full time, on top of juggling family and social responsibilities. Because they don't "work out for a living," as some of them say, they often fit in far fewer workouts than they'd like. One client confessed, "I think of myself as such an active person, but the truth is, it's more wishful thinking than reality." And one of the biggest problems with overestimating how much you exercise is misjudging how much food you need, which can be a top barrier to seeing results.

This is one of the reasons why I chose to designate starchy foods as "energy accessories" to be tacked on to meals in quantities that match your body's needs, which can change from day to day or even within one day (see page 87 to determine how to adjust your meals in this way). It's also why the movement plan in chapter 8 is designed to help you overcome the biggest barriers to being active and to find ways to be physical you can squeeze into even the busiest days. Bottom line: getting real about how active you are can prevent you from eating meals, even healthy ones, that contain surpluses that feed fat you want to shed.

Attending Get-Togethers and Holiday Celebrations

When you're on a quest to shed pounds, getting through a holiday can feel like navigating an obstacle course. Most of my clients are part of social circles where it's normal to overeat or eat decadent or processed foods. One of my clients described going to watch a big football game at a friend's home, where the only foods available were pizza, wings, chips and dip, candy, brownies, soda, and alcohol. Though she knew she wouldn't be facing a display of health-food fare, she had hoped for a lighter option, like a veggie tray or fresh fruit. She did the best she could, sticking to a few slices of cheese pizza and a light beer. But she left feeling bloated, unsatisfied, and disappointed that she didn't think to eat before the party or bring food with her. On top of that, she felt that the pizza, which wasn't from her favorite pizzeria, wasn't worth the splurge. To avoid this kind of dietary disappointment, put the following four strategies into action the next time you're invited to a social gathering or holiday dinner.

Bring a healthy dish or two.

It's perfectly okay to bring healthy fare to a get-together, as long as you bring enough to share. You can take along foods that cover the meal staples in this plan (lean protein, veggies, and plant-based fat) and even the pulse or other energy accessory if you'd like. Great options include shrimp cocktail or grilled chicken skewers for lean protein and raw or roasted and chilled veggies with guacamole for veggies and plant-based fat. Party-friendly energy accessories include popcorn, fresh-cut fruit, chilled lentil salad, roasted chickpeas, bean dip, and hummus. Filling your plate with this healthy fare will easily allow you to take smaller portions of, or even skip, the heavy stuff.

Pick a starch—one starch.

Carb overload is usually the reason you feel heavier or your jeans feel snug after a holiday or get-together. That's why I've paid such careful attention to energy accessories in this plan. When you think about it, most of what we enjoy in special occasion meals is laden with starch. You don't have to give up carbs completely to lose weight, but preventing carb overload is key. So if you opt for an energy accessory that's more of a splurge, like a slice of pie, use my How to Squeeze in a Splurge tips on page 301 to keep things in balance.

Rethink your drinks.

If you'll be toasting the holiday or occasion, use my tips starting on page 283 to prevent a cocktail or two from triggering a feeding frenzy.

Build in postmeal activity.

If you do wind up enjoying a cupcake or dipping into the M&M dish, grab a friend or family member you'd like to catch up with and take a fifteen-minute walk. In addition to balancing out your extras, this technique can help normalize your blood sugar levels for up to three hours after eating, research shows, even if you're walking at an easy-to-moderate pace. If the weather is too chilly to get outside, find fun ways to move indoors. Play an active game, like Wii, organize an old-school game of charades, or just visit with someone special as you tackle the dishes together. Even just standing burns 50 percent more calories than sitting.

Dining Out

Dining at a restaurant tends to be a high-risk occasion for many of my clients, because they feel tempted to order foods that don't fit into the plan, like a mile-high slice of meaty lasagna, or because ordering from a menu can feel overwhelming. Here are strategies to help you overcome restaurant temptations.

Connect the dots between your choices and the outcomes.

By keeping food journals, one of my clients discovered that she nearly always eats from her husband's and children's plates, especially when dining out. When we talked about why—what she was thinking and feeling when she found herself doing this—she realized it was because it was a way of cheating. She could sneak fries or ice cream from her kids' plates without feeling as guilty as if she had ordered French fries or an ice cream–covered skillet cookie herself. But the sneaking left her feeling overly full and sluggish after meals, and she wasn't hungry when it was time to eat again. As a result, she was not losing weight. Because the extras were stealthy, she hadn't really identified this habit as the culprit, but when we talked about the pros and cons of continuing the pattern, it hit her like a ton of bricks that she had really been cheating herself. She renewed her commitment to using the techniques, like the splurge strategy on page 301, that she knew worked, and she started back on a losing path. If dining out is a challenge for you, revisit the reasons you set out on this journey.

Order unapologetically.

These days, customizing your order when dining out is the norm, and in my experience, it's a habit shared by people who stay slim without "dieting." Naturally slim people modify their orders not to lose weight but to eat in a way that makes them feel well. I waited tables all through college and grad school, and I remember one regular customer who, long before white hamburger buns were considered evil, always ordered her turkey burgers bunless. She'd say, "If I have that bun, I won't have room for popcorn at the movies," or "If I eat that bun, I'll feel like taking a nap rather than shopping!" To her, ditching the bun wasn't about dieting; it just made sense. You can adopt the same approach when you select your meals. Refer to the list of restaurant options that fit the wardrobe design on page 172, and use these basic tips when dining out:

- Eat your energy accessory, such as 1 cup of grapes, ½ cup of Oven-Roasted Chickpeas, or a serving of whole-grain crackers, before you head to the restaurant. This tactic can help prevent you from being overly hungry when you order and reduce the chances that you'll overdo it with an oversize portion of brown rice or potatoes.

- At a sushi place, meet the wardrobe design with
  Lean protein: seared tuna or sashimi
  Veggies: steamed broccoli or a side salad
  Plant-based fat: avocado

- At a Mexican place, meet the wardrobe design with
  Lean protein: grilled chicken or shrimp or black beans
  Veggies: a salad dressed with pico de gallo or salsa
  Plant-based fat: avocado or guacamole

- At a seafood place, meet the wardrobe design with
  Lean protein: grilled or broiled fish or shrimp cocktail
  Veggies: steamed, sautéed, or grilled vegetables or a side salad
  Plant-based fat: olive oil for the salad (with vinegar, fresh lemon, and cracked black pepper), or oil may already be in the grilled or sautéed veggies

No Time to Spare

Time constraints can make it challenging to prioritize healthy eating. If you're worn out after a long day, thinking about what to make for dinner can feel like a major burden. And without healthy options in place, it's easy to order takeout or reach for processed snacks or comfort foods. But having healthy options at the ready doesn't have to be a time suck. Here are five tips that really work for my time-challenged clients and for me.

Opt for a grab-and-go grocery meal.

Forget the drive-through! Instead, pop into a supermarket and head for the prepared foods section. Grab grilled salmon or chicken for lean protein, and a chilled vegetable salad, which can fill the veggie and plant-based fat components of the wardrobe design. Zip through the express line, and you'll be back in your car as quickly as if you'd ordered from a drive-through.

Keep go-to meal staples on hand.

In chapter 5, I noted which meals are quick, which means they can be made in twenty minutes or less. Choose a few of these meals and stock up on the ingredients so you'll always be able to whip up a few easy meals in a jiffy.

Stash made-ahead meals in the fridge or freezer.

In chapter 5, I indicated which meals can be made ahead and which can be frozen and reheated. On days when you have extra time, perhaps Sundays, choose a few meals to prep and store, so they're ready to eat, or heat and eat, when you need them.

Cobble together snacks that make a meal.

It may not be the most gourmet choice, but in a pinch, combining simple, plain foods like the following can fill the diet wardrobe design and get you through:

- *Lean proteins:* thawed frozen cooked shrimp; chunk light tuna canned in water; grilled chicken breast; hard-boiled eggs; precooked, vacuum-sealed lentils
- *Veggies:* raw veggies, ready-to-eat salad greens, steamed fresh or frozen veggies
- *Plant-based fats:* nuts or seeds, olives or olive tapenade; pesto; avocado or premade all-natural guacamole

Whip up a meal.

Smoothies aren't just for breakfast. Since all the meals in my plan are interchangeable, you can enjoy any of the smoothies in chapter 5 as breakfast, lunch, or dinner. Blending one and taking it with you can be a great way to save time.

Losing Motivation

We all have days when we just want to say "Screw it!" and order a pizza, crack open a bottle of wine, and give in to what feels good right now. But in all my years of counseling clients, I've never come across anyone who hasn't lamented giving up. The temporary bliss is followed by days of feeling bloated, heavy, and full of regret. Even clients who've said to me "Maybe I'll just accept being fat" don't really want to embrace that prospect; it's just their emotions talking in the moment. So many things, from a rough day at work to a challenging day of parenting, or even a rude store clerk, can trigger the "screw it" switch. When your mind goes there, put the following tactics into action.

Remember your goals.

One of the reasons you took on my challenge was because you wanted to feel good physically and emotionally. You chose this plan, rather than another more extreme or restrictive "quick fix" approach to weight loss, because energy, wellness, and good health are important and meaningful to you. Remind yourself that giving up would mean sacrificing those aspirations.

Shift your mind-set.

Simply believing you can change your habits and routines can help you do just that. In a recent study that analyzed the diets, exercise habits, and personality types of more than seven thousand people, those who believed they could change their lives through their own actions ate more healthfully, exercised more, and were less likely to drink too much and smoke. When clients tell me "I'll never be able to change," I ask them to name something else they changed or achieved that they felt doubtful about but were able to ultimately accomplish, and they can always think of something. Reminding yourself of your past successes can help shift your mind-set and allow you to feel more confident about your ability to transform your lifestyle today.

Re-read chapter 7.

I've read sections of some self-help books dozens of times. Though you may know the content in chapter 7, reading it again can help the information sink in or click in a new way, or help you refocus on your mediation practice. I firmly believe that meditating regularly is an integral part of this plan, because losing weight for good goes far beyond just knowing what to eat. Meditation can transform your mind-set, allow you to react to situations in a completely different way, and keep you focused on your goals.

Travel

I travel a lot, and though airports offer many more healthy options than they used to, I pack my own foods as a backup or supplement, so I won't be at the mercy of what's available in the terminal. Here are my go-to options and strategies.

Task 1: build the wardrobe.

At any airport, I can usually find healthy, lean protein options, even pulses, like a side of black beans, chickpeas, or vegetarian refried beans, without the cheese. At LAX I always order a terrific veggie and bean chili, and at JFK I can get my standard salad topped with chickpeas or black beans. While both of these already come with veggies, I always bring extras, like grape tomatoes, red bell pepper sliced into strips, or fresh snow peas. For plant-based fat, I pack nuts. When I order a salad, if I can't get avocado, I'll add my own nuts. And rather than using dressing, I'll ask for a side of plain balsamic vinegar and mix in a packet of mustard. It's so flavorful and it perfectly coats the veggies, so I can forego premade pouches, which are typically laden with sugar, sodium, and artificial additives.

Task 2: tack on an energy accessory.

Though most airports sell fruit, it can be expensive and not so stellar in quality, so I bring my own. Seedless grapes are my favorite. But there are plenty of nonperishable energy accessory choices that travel well, including whole-grain crackers and prepopped popcorn.

Task 3: stock my hotel room.

The first thing I do if I can is find the nearest grocery or health-food store, so I have plenty of choices while I'm in town. For example, if I go out to dinner and there are no nutritious energy accessory options on the menu, I'll eat fresh fruit when I get back to my room. I also pack extra zip-top plastic bags so I can bring healthy fare with me on my flight home.

Lack of Support

Numerous clients have told me that when they turn down food or drinks, friends and family members make comments like "You don't need to lose weight—you look fine." Many report feeling guilted into eating foods

• •

THE TRUTH ABOUT HOLIDAY WEIGHT GAIN

A study from Texas Tech University followed nearly 150 men and women for the six weeks between Thanksgiving and New Year's Day. On average, the men gained about two pounds each and the women gained one pound, far less than the seven to ten pounds often cited as typical weight gain during the holidays. One to two pounds might not sound like much, but the trouble is, we tend to not lose that holiday weight. That's what leads most Americans to pack on ten to twenty pounds per decade, typically referred to as "weight creep."

• •

they're trying to avoid. Research shows that, bullied or not, friends who eat together eat more food than those paired with strangers, and friends give each other "permission" to overeat. To break the cycle, try these five approaches.

Break the eating-as-entertainment pattern.

Rather than scheduling social time around happy hours and dinners out, change up how you spend time with the people you care about. For example, instead of going to a movie, go to a play, where munching on popcorn and candy isn't allowed.

Explain your motives.

If your friends and family push back, explain that you're on a health quest that goes beyond weight loss. Let them know that eating better helps you sleep better and puts you in a better mood, so you're more productive at work and even-tempered with your kids. Or maybe healthier living keeps your heartburn and migraines at bay. Once others understand that you're not just aiming to become a smaller size, they may have more respect for your efforts.

Confront thoughtfully.

Confrontation is never comfortable, but being honest about how you feel may be the only way to work through this issue. Approach the situation gently. Rather than attack or accuse, take your friends or family members aside, let them know that the relationship is important you, and ask for their support.

See things through their eyes.

Typically, a lack of support is really more about your friend or family member than you. Your healthy efforts may trigger others to feel guilty about overindulging themselves or force them to take a look at unhealthy habits they aren't ready to face. Or the resistance may stem from a loving place. After all, many of us are socialized to believe that food represents affection. Try to understand where your loved one is coming from. You may be surprised to learn that comments you're perceiving as unsupportive are not at all spiteful.

Find cheerleaders elsewhere.

Even online "friends" you'll never meet, who share your interests and goals, can be a great group to rely on. Having even one person in your corner who "gets it" can give you the confidence and motivation you need to deal with challenging situations.

HOW TO SQUEEZE IN A SPLURGE

This may be one of the most important sections in this book, because at some point, you're going to want to eat a can't-live-without food that doesn't neatly fit into this plan. If I can show you how to do that without deviating too much from the wardrobe design, you can literally have your cake (or French fries or ice cream) and eat it too. Here's how to do it in four steps.

Zero in on your target.

Many of my clients find themselves eating food they don't even really like, simply because it's there. These second-rate splurges aren't very satisfying and can actually drive a craving rather than squelch one. That's why it's important to splurge only on foods you absolutely love. If a treat is tempting you, rate it using a five-star scale, five being "Can't-live-without, 100 percent worthwhile," and zero being "Meh, if I pass it up, I won't feel deprived." If a food rates a three or less, skip it. You may find it helpful to make a list of your favorites, foods you know you simply cannot or don't want to swear off forever. If your instinct is to say "I don't want to eat any bad foods anymore," remember that long-term weight control is a lifetime commitment, and never having certain foods ever again just isn't realistic for most of us.

Opt out to add in.

If your chosen splurge contains carbs, omit the energy accessory in your meal to make room for them. If your chosen treat also contains fat, omit that as well. You'll find fat in most carb-rich splurges, including potato chips, cheese, and cupcakes. But if you're craving something that's all sugar with little fat, like jelly beans or gummy candies, leave the plant-based fat in your meal. This means your meal should consist of a serving of lean protein, one to two servings of veggies, and possibly the plant-based fat, depending on your splurge. For example, one of my clients loved holiday-themed candies, like message hearts around Valentine's Day, marshmallow chicks at Easter, and fun-size candy bars around Halloween. Her typical lunch was a few cups of greens and veggies, tossed with balsamic vinegar, a squeeze of fresh lemon, and cracked black pepper, and topped with 3 ounces of chunk light tuna. When she incorporated the hearts or marshmallow chicks, she added avocado to the salad, but when she went for mini candy bars made with chocolate and nuts, she left the avocado off. If your chosen splurge is a protein that's not so lean, such as cheese or red meat, omit the fat in the meal and leave in the veggies and energy accessory. For example, enjoy an ounce of hard cheese with roasted vegetables and whole-grain crackers. Or eat a small filet along with steamed broccoli and oven-roasted red potatoes.

Select a "not my last hurrah" portion.

Nearly all of my clients who have tried to lose weight in the past have binged on "forbidden foods" either before starting a "diet" or after falling off one. The fact is, an all-or-nothing mentality is guaranteed to set you up for failure. In that mind-set, one splurge triggers thoughts like "I'm not going to be able to have this, so I better get as much as I can now" or "Well, I blew it, I might as well go all out." Those extremes will keep you stuck. In fact, failing to build in indulgences is the primary reason many people ride the weight roller coaster—lose 20 pounds, gain back 25, lose 30, gain back 40, and so on. When you try to be "perfect" week after week, you'll likely end up with pent-up feelings of deprivation, resentment, or even anger or depression. Ultimately, you'll binge. As a nutritionist, I'm never, ever going to say that a donut is healthy. However, I've been in practice long enough to know that when people swear off foods they can't or aren't ready to give up, they either overeat other foods in an attempt to get that fix or they eventually give in and binge on the forbidden food. Then they feel stuffed, sluggish, and remorseful. That's why, on my plan, no food on the planet is off-limits. It makes far more sense to enjoy decadent foods using a strategy to keep them in balance. (Remember the debt analogy I described on page 64?) You can splurge every single week if you'd like (up to two meals a week on nonconsecutive days, as I noted on page 202), so there's no need to feel like you have to eat a giant portion when you do. If you're eating a packaged food, aim to stick with the serving size listed. If you're ordering ice cream, opt for a small rather than a medium or large. Just knowing you can have that same treat again within a week or less should allow you to feel like it's okay to go easy.

Savor every morsel.

When you enjoy any splurge, make it special. You've chosen a food that's completely worthwhile, and you've opted to remove other foods from your meal to make room for your treat. Make it even more special by eating it without the distraction of TV or your computer. Take your time, and pay attention to the aroma, flavor, and texture of your indulgence. This awareness can significantly boost your enjoyment and trigger satiety hormones, which help you feel content with a reasonable portion. If you hit that mark before the treat is gone, you don't have to finish it. Work on stopping when you feel like you've had enough, tossing the rest, and moving on.

If you're worried that you won't be able to control your portion size, wait to splurge until you feel ready. Or allow yourself to splurge in ways that reduce your chances of overeating. For example, once a week, split a dessert at a restaurant or buy one cookie from a bakery rather than bringing home a box. If you don't have leftovers, you won't be tempted to eat more. For more about splurging, including an exercise that can help you differentiate a craving for a specific food from emotionally triggered eating, see page 289.

Acknowledgments

To everyone at HarperCollins—thank you for the opportunity to share this book with the world. Special thanks to Mark Tauber for your support, Suzanne Wickham for being such a dream to work with, and my editor, Nancy Hancock, for your faith in my professional philosophies and practice, our talks about life and our pets, and for honoring my voice in this book. And thanks to Gideon Weil for jumping in and being so terrific to work with.

To my agent, Richard Abate—thank you for believing in me, being on my side, your awesome sense of humor, and for always being available when I need you. I feel incredibly grateful to be working with you. And huge appreciation to the amazing Marta Tracy of Marty Tracy Entertainment. Thank you for your tireless, passionate work, incredible loyalty, generosity, and friendship. I feel so lucky to have found you.

This book could not have come together without the talents and support of Suzanne Scholsberg and McKenzie Hall. I can't thank you enough for your help, professionalism, and feedback. I hope you know how much I admire you both professionally and personally.

Thank you to Kristina Nicole Mallon and Kelly Sloan, dietetic students when you volunteered your time and skills to help me with this project. I'm excited to watch your careers unfold. I have no doubt that each of you will succeed in anything you set out to do, and I am thrilled to be your colleague.

To all of my clients—thank you for putting your trust in me and making me feel like I truly have a dream job. And to the incredible women who made the commitment to formally test this eating plan. It was such an honor and a privilege to get to know each of you. Your invaluable feedback and experiences have improved this book, and your stories are truly inspirational. I feel like we bonded for life over pulses, and I look forward to keeping in touch!

Many thanks to everyone at *Health* magazine, especially Clare McHugh, Lisa Lombardi, Theresa Tamkins, Susan Rinkunas, Amelia Harnish, Caitlin Eadie, Erin Clinton, and MaryAnn Barone. I love being part of the *Health* family. I admire all you do to help women across the country live healthier, happier lives.

Much appreciation to my trusted friends, who have always lent their support and encouragement, especially Lynn Miller, Jackie Newgent, Rachel Meltzer Warren, Leah McLaughlin, James Corbett, Brittany Doyle and Tom Hanc, Jennifer Cohen, McKenzie Hall, and Tara Gidus. I'm so lucky to have all of you in my life.

To my parents, James and Carol Crowell, and every member of my Crowell, Sass, DeTota, Miller, and Salvagno families—I love you all so much. Very special thanks to my brother Steve Crowell, sister Diane Salvagno, and "sister" Lynn Miller for really being there for me during a particularly challenging time this year—I'm so grateful.

And finally to my husband, Jack Bremen, and my amazing sister Diane Salvagno, to whom this book is dedicated. Jack, you are *always* there for me. You've been my rock through every step of this journey. You've stepped up to help me with everything from concept and writing feedback to taste testing, tech support, photography, and moral support. Thank you for making me feel loved, making me laugh, helping me find balance, and bringing out the best in me. And to Diane—even though we live miles apart I feel like we couldn't be closer. Thank you for honest feedback and support, unconditional love, friendship, and laughter.

Selected Bibliography

Abete, I., D. Parra, and J. Martinez. "Legume-, Fish-, or High-Protein-Based Hypocaloric Diets: Effects on Weight Loss and Mitochondrial Oxidation in Obese Men." *Journal of Medicinal Food* 12, no. 1 (2009): 100–8. http://online.liebertpub.com/doi/abs/10.1089/jmf.2007.0700.

Bazzano, L., J. He, L. Ogden, C. Loria, S. Vupputuri, L. Myers, and P. Whelton. "Legume Consumption and Risk of Coronary Heart Disease in U.S. Men and Women." *Archives of Internal Medicine* 161, no. 21 (2001): 2573–78. http://archinte.jamanetwork.com/article.aspx?articleid=649612.

Bourdon, I., B. Olson, R. Backus, B. Richter, P. Davis, and B. Schneeman. "Beans, as a Source of Dietary Fiber, Increase Cholecystokinin and Apolipoprotein b48 Response to Test Meals in Men." *Journal of Nutrition* 131, no. 5 (2001): 1485–90.

Camara, C. R., C. A. Urrea, and V. Schlegel. "Pinto Beans (*Phaseolus Vulgaris* L.) as a Functional Food: Implications on Human Heath." *Agriculture* 3, no. 1 (2013): 90–111.

Diepvens, K., D. Häberer, and M. Westerterp-Plantenga. "Different Proteins and Biopeptides Differently Affect Satiety and Anorexigenic/Orexigenic Hormones in Healthy Humans." *International Journal of Obesity (London)* 32, no. 3 (2008): 510–18. http://www.ncbi.nlm.nih.gov/pubmed/18345020.

Drewnowski, A., and C. Rehm. "Vegetable Cost Metrics Show That Potatoes and Beans Provide Most Nutrients Per Penny." *PLoS ONE* 8, no. 5 (2013): e63277. http://www.plosone.org/article/info%3Adoi%2F10.1371%2Fjournal.pone.0063277.

Farvid, M., E. Cho, W. Chen, A. Eliassen, and W. Willett. "Dietary Protein Sources in Early Adulthood and Breast Cancer Incidence: Prospective Cohort Study." *British Medical Journal* 338 (2014): 3437. http://www.ncbi.nlm.nih.gov/pmc/articles/PMC4051890/.

Forster, G., C. Ollila, J. Burton, D. Hill, J. Bauer, A. Hess, and E. Ryan. "Nutritional Weight Loss Therapy with Cooked Bean Powders Regulates Serum Lipids and Biochemical Analytes in Overweight and Obese Dogs." *Journal of Obesity and Weight Loss Therapy* 2, no. 8 (2012): 1–8. http://csu-cvmbs.colostate.edu/Documents/erhs-weightloss-and-bean-canine-eryan-lab.pdf.

Hairston, K., M. Vitolins, J. Norris, A. Anderson, A. Hanley, and L. Wagenknecht. "Lifestyle Factors and 5-Year Abdominal Fat Accumulation in a Minority Cohort: The IRAS Family Study." *Obesity (Silver Spring)* 20, no. 2 (2012): 421–27. http://www.ncbi.nlm.nih.gov/pubmed/21681224.

Hairston, K., M. Vitolins, J. Norris, A. Anderson, A. Hanley, and L. Wagenknecht. "Soluble Fiber Strikes a Blow to Belly Fat." Wake Forest Baptist Medical Center. ScienceDaily (June 27, 2011). Accessed October 8, 2014. http://www.science-daily.com/releases/2011/06/110627123032.htm.

Hermsdorff, H., M. Zulet, I. Abete, and J. Martinez. "A Legume-Based Hypocaloric Diet Reduces Pro-Inflammatory Status and Improves Metabolic Features in Overweight/Obese Subjects." *European Journal of Nutrition* 50, no. 1 (2011): 61–69. http://www.ncbi.nlm.nih.gov/pubmed/20499072.

Jenkins, D., C. Kendall, L. Augustin, S. Mitchell, S. Sahye-Pudaruth, S. Blanco Mejia, L. Chiavaroli, et al. "Effect of Legumes as Part of a Low Glycemic Index Diet on Glycemic Control and Cardiovascular Risk Factors in Type 2 Diabetes Mellitus: A Randomized Controlled Trial." *Archives of Internal Medicine* 172, no. 21 (2012): 1653–60. http://www.ncbi.nlm.nih.gov/pubmed/23089999.

Karamanolis, I., K. Laparidis, K. Volaklis, H. Douda, and S. Tokmakidis. "The Effects of Pre-Exercise Glycemic Index Food on Running Capacity." *International Journal of Sports Medicine* 32, no. 9 (2011): 666–71.

Lanza, E., T. J. Hartman, P. S. Albert, R. Shields, M. Slattery, B. Saen, E. Paskett, et al. "High Dry Bean Intake and Reduced Risk of Advanced Colorectal Adenoma Recurrence Among Participants in the Polyp Prevention Trial." *Journal of Nutrition* 136, no. 7 (2006): 1896–903.

Leatherwood, P., and P. Pollet. "Effects of Slow Release Carbohydrates in the Form of Bean Flakes on the Evolution of Hunger and Satiety in Man." *Appetite* 10, no. 1 (1988): 1–11.

Marinangeli, C. P., and P. J. Jones. "Pulse Grain Consumption and Obesity: Effects on Energy Expenditure, Substrate Oxidation, Body Composition, Fat Deposition, and Satiety." *British Journal of Nutrition* 108, suppl. 1 (2012): S46–51.

Marinangeli, C. P., and P. J. Jones. "Whole and Fractionated Yellow Pea Flours Reduce Fasting Insulin and Insulin Resistance in Hypercholesterolaemic and Overweight Human Subjects." *British Journal of Nutrition* 105, no. 1 (2011): 110–17. http://journals.cambridge.org/action/displayAbstract?fromPage=online&aid=7948474&fileId=S0007114510003156.

Marinangeli, C. P., D. Krause, S. V. Harding, T. C. Rideout, F. Zhu, and P. J. Jones. "Whole and Fractionated Yellow Pea Flours Modulate Insulin, Glucose, Oxygen Consumption, and the Caecal Microbiome in Golden Syrian Hamsters." *Applied Physiology, Nutrition, and Metabolism* 36, no. 6 (2011): 811–20. http://www.ingentaconnect.com/content/nrc/apnm/2011/00000036/00000006/art00005.

McCrory, M., J. Lovejoy, P. Palmer, P. Eichelsdoerfer, M. Gehrke, I. Kavanaugh, S. Buesing, and T. Rose. "Effectiveness of Legume Consumption for Facilitating Weight Loss: A Randomized Trial." *FASEB Journal* 22 (2008): 1084–89. http://www.fasebj.org/cgi/content/meeting_abstract/22/1_MeetingAbstracts/1084.8.

Mollard, R., B. Luhovyy, S. Panahi, M. Nunez, A. Hanley, and G. Anderson. "Regular Consumption of Pulses for 8 Weeks Reduces Metabolic Syndrome Risk Factors in Overweight and Obese Adults." *British Journal of Nutrition* 108 (2012): s111–22. http://journals.cambridge.org/download.php?file=%2FBJN%2FBJN108_S1%2FS0007114512000712a.pdf&code=864 38f875dcaac3e215d621ee092fd38.

Mudryi, A. N., N. Yu, and H. M. Aukema. "Nutritional and Health Benefits of Pulses." *Applied Physiology, Nutrition, and Metabolism* 39, no. 11 (2014): 1197–204.

Mudryi, A. N., N. Yu, T. J. Hartman, D. C. Mitchell, F. R. Lawrence, and H. M. Aukema. "Pulse Consumption in Canadian Adults Influences Nutrient Intakes." *British Journal of Nutrition* 108, suppl. 1 (2012): S27–36.

Murty, C., J. Pittaway, and M. Ball. "Chickpea Supplementation in an Australian Diet Affects Food Choice, Satiety, and Bowel Health." *Appetite* 54, no. 2 (2010): 282–88. http://www.ncbi.nlm.nih.gov/pubmed/19945492.

"'Musical Fruit' Rich Source of Healthy Antioxidants; Black Beans Highest." *American Chemical Society* (December 3, 2003). Accessed October 8, 2014. http://www.eurekalert.org/pub_releases/2003-12/acs-fr120303.php.

"Research Shows Adults and Teens Who Eat Beans Weigh Less." From the National Nutrition and Health Examination Survey. National Center for Health Statistics. April 3, 2006. Accessed October 8, 2014. http://www.eurekalert.org/pub_releases/2006-04/epr-rsa033106.php.

Tachibana, N., S. Wanezaki, M. Nagata, T. Motoyama, M. Kohno, and S. Kitagawa. "Intake of Mung Bean Protein Isolate Reduces Plasma Triglyceride Level in Rats." *Functional Foods in Health and Disease* 3, no. 9 (2013): 365–76.

Thompson, M. D., M. A. Brick, J. N. McGinley, and H. J. Thompson. "Chemical Composition and Mammary Cancer Inhibitory Activity of Dry Bean." *Crop Science* 49, no. 1 (2009): 179–86.

Tonstad, S., N. Mailk, and E. Haddad. "A High-Fibre Bean-Rich Diet Versus a Low-Carbohydrate Diet for Obesity." *Journal of Human Nutrition and Dietetics* 27, no. s2 (2013): 109–16.

Windham, D., and A. Hutchins. "Perceptions of Flatulence from Bean Consumption Among Adults in 3 Feeding Studies." *Nutrition Journal* 10, no. 1 (2011): 128. http://www.nutritionj.com/content/10/1/128.

Yang, Y., L. Zhou, Y. Gu, Y. Zhang, J. Tang, F. Li, W. Shang, B. Jiang, X. Yue, and M. Chen. "Dietary Chickpeas Reverse Visceral Adiposity Dyslipidaemia and Insulin Resistance in Rats Induced by a Chronic High-Fat Diet." *British Journal of Nutrition* 98, no. 4 (2007): 720–26. http://journals.cambridge.org/action/displayAbstract?fromPage=online&aid=1343196&fileId=S0007114507750870.

Index

About the Author

Cynthia Sass is skilled in nearly every facet of nutrition and health communications—as a *New York Times* bestselling author, magazine columnist and editor, blogger, freelance writer, keynote speaker, contributor to a national news network, and regular national television guest, as well as as a practitioner, with nearly two decades of experience.

Cynthia graduated with highest honors from Syracuse University, where she earned a bachelor's degree in dietetics, followed by a master's degree in nutrition science, with a concentration in counseling. She completed a second master's degree in public health at the University of South Florida, one of only forty nationally accredited colleges of public health in the country, with a concentration in community and family-health education. Sass also completed a personal-trainer certification at the Cooper Institute for Aerobics Research in Dallas, Texas, and plant-based organic culinary arts training at the Institute for Culinary Awakening in Portland, Oregon.

One of the first registered dietitians to become board certified as a specialist in sports dietetics, Sass is in her fifth season as the sports nutrition consultant to the New York Rangers, and in her eighth season with the Tampa Bay Rays. Sass also served as the nutrition consultant to the Philadelphia Phillies from 2007 to 2009. She proudly rooted for both the Rays and the Phillies (at the time she was a consultant for both teams) as they faced each other in the 2008 World Series.

Cynthia has been in private practice for nearly twenty years, counseling a wide range of clients, including professional athletes in numerous sports, actors, musicians, fashion models, CEOs, new moms, teens, couples, and families. She is also the consulting nutritionist for UCLA's prestigious executive health program.

A go-to resource for the media, Cynthia has appeared on *The Today Show, Good Morning America, CBS This Morning,* the *Rachael Ray Show, The Dr. Oz. Show, The Doctors, The Biggest Loser, Nightline, The Martha Stewart Show,* CNN, *Access Hollywood Live,* ABC's *World News Tonight,* and many other national programs. She was an ABC News on-air contributor from 2009 to 2011.

Cynthia is currently a contributing editor at *Health* magazine and blogger for Health.com. She was a contributing editor, columnist, and blogger at *Shape* magazine from 2008 to 2012, and previously served as the nutrition director at *Prevention* magazine. She is also currently a contributing editor, columnist, and the sole nutritionist for *Athletes Quarterly,* an exclusive publication for and about professional athletes.

Cynthia's last book, *S.A.S.S. Yourself Slim: Conquer Cravings, Drop Pounds, and Lose Inches* (formerly published as *Cinch!: Conquer Cravings, Drop Pounds, and Lose Inches*), debuted at #3 on the January 23, 2011, *New York Times* bestsellers list and has remained popular due to its simple, effective, flexible, and sustainable weight-loss approach. Previously, Cynthia cowrote the #1 *New York Times* bestselling book *Flat Belly Diet!,* and she is the creator of its deliciously slimming eating plan. She also coauthored the *Flat Belly Diet! Cookbook,* another *New York Times* bestseller. Additionally Sass is the coauthor of the unique personalized food journal entitled *The Ultimate Diet Log,* as well as the relationship book *Your Diet Is Driving Me Crazy: When Food Conflicts Get in the*

Way of Your Love Life, which received a glowing review in the *New York Times* and was a finalist in the relationship category of the 2004 Books for a Better Life Awards.

Huffington Post named Cynthia one of thirty-five diet and nutrition experts you need to follow on Twitter. She tweets @CynthiaSass, where she regularly leads live chats for @goodhealth with the hashtag #Talk Nutrition. To learn more about Cynthia and access her weekly blogs, visit www.CynthiaSass.com.